30 Days to A Vibrant, Healthier, Younger You

Tomasa Macapinlac

This book may be purchased for educational, business or sales promotional use. For more information, please email: info@selfcarequeendom.com.

ISBN-10: 1-5375068-3-8

ISBN-13: 978-1-5375068-3-8

Library of Congress Number: 2016921054

The author of this book does not dispense medical advice or prescribe the use of any technique as a form of treatment for physical, emotional, or medical problems without the advice of a physician, either directly or indirectly. The ideas, procedures, and suggestions contained in this book are intended to complement the advice of your healthcare provider, not replace it. All matters regarding your health require medical supervision. The intent of the author is only to offer information of a general nature to help you in your quest for emotional and spiritual well-being. In the event you use any of the information in this book for yourself, which is your constitutional right, the author and the publisher assume no responsibility for your actions.

Contents

Dedication

This book is dedicated to all my current and past clients, students, friends and family members who have helped me to articulate in written form what I have shared with you in other ways. I thank you all for the encouragement to write even when I kept on insisting that it was too big of a project for me to share in written form. And thank you to my senior clients who encouraged me that my information needed to be in book form as the virtual video version was not a medium that they were used to accessing in their lifetime. So ta da.. here's the written version.

Introduction

I am writing this book to encourage all women to consciously embrace the aging process, whether they be busy moms, 40- to 50-year-old women wondering how all the years of fatigue may be showing up on their faces, or senior women over 60 who want to stay active regardless of how their bodies might be telling them to slow down.

You see, in my early thirties, I started receiving ancient healing methods to bring myself back from fatigue and a compromised immune system (which happens when your children go to daycare and preschool and expose you to all of their germs). Oh, but wait, I was supposed to be this "supermom" who could combat anything with her mind, right? Sometimes your body feels like an old car that hasn't been maintained with a simple oil change every 5,000 miles.

It took me crashing and burning with my own energy reserves to really wake up and see what was really going on with me. In 1996, I had this picture perfect family. A family of four, we were living in the greater suburbs of the San Francisco Bay Area. Let me paint a picture for you – I was dressing for success, going to work in name-brand suits and pumps I bought from Nordstrom's or Macy's, doing whatever it took to make the almighty dollar so I could support what I thought was an ideal, holistic, SUCCESSFUL lifestyle of organic foods and private Montessori schooling for my two toddler daughters. Although it seemed like I had a lot of energy, it was superficial energy that was unfocused and scattered, making it hard for me to complete tasks.

On the outside, I looked great. How I felt on the inside was a different story. There was no end to the madness of the rat race. The soles of my feet burned. My shoulder blades were always tense. After picking up my daughters from day care, feeding them and sometimes having conference calls with the factory and customers well after a good day of work, I would fall asleep at 9 pm.

Everyone thinks the life of a sales executive is all about fine dining with customers, jetsetting to customer and factory sites or golfing with your customers to close million dollar deals. But let me tell you that while I enjoyed traveling to different places and lunching with my customers, at home I got to decompress and unsuppress the agonizing pain, which made me constantly wonder if life was going to continue this way. I used to love shopping, but I simply couldn't do it anymore because my feet ached all the time. I didn't even want to go out on the weekends and do fun things with my girls – I just wanted to rest up so I could be ready for work the following week. And yes, there was little physical intimacy shared with my partner at the time... who had the energy for that?

Finally, one day, it hit me like a ton of bricks. I was awakened by the aches and pains of the common cold, but this time was different – I was exhausted. Utterly and completely exhausted. So exhausted that I couldn't even get good rest. Have you ever been there?

I would go to work and by noon, I just wanted to go back to

bed. I didn't even know how I was going to drive myself home because I didn't have the energy at all. You know how you keep thinking that you're going to get better if you just wait it out? Well, I kept thinking and hoping that this would be the case, but somehow I ended up in my MD's office.

She told me to just go home and get bed rest for 3 days without doing anything. I was forbidden from taking care of my girls, cleaning, working, or even cooking. Lucky me, I thought. Yes, I was finally getting a vacation from all my Chief of the Household duties. I followed orders, and after 3 days, I was still tired, hopeless and worried about what was happening to my 32-year-old self. In a month I would turn 33, and I didn't understand what had hit me.

A co-worker (now a client) came to the rescue and gave me the name and number of a holistic practitioner who she thought could help. I carried that number in my purse for a few days, hoping I would get better. Finally, I caved in and called the practitioner.

When I got on the table to receive these ancient healing modalities, I had no idea that I would experience what I did. Not only did my body feel much better, but I felt like someone had plugged me into Source, Spirit or the Universe. I had been Robot Mom, wife and fast-track hi-tech sales executive, so focused on taking care of my customers and family that I forgot to take care of the most important person: myself. That day of receiving such ancient healing touched my life forever, and it has been the turning point in how I take care of myself. I learned not only how to work on myself, but I went on to learn how to work with others as well so that no one would have to experience what I did.

Even though I am no longer in the corporate world, the world of an entrepreneur is just as demanding; the key difference is that it's within my control and I get to do work that I love. In fact, it's that very love of what I'm doing that keeps me ticking, helps me focus when I need to complete a task that might not be my genius, and lifts me up when I need that extra boost to complete a project – because let me tell you, entrepreneurship is no piece of cake.

What I've learned is, you can't numb out like you can in the corporate world – you certainly feel everything you are going through, better known as the fast track to personal growth. There can be emotional ups and downs as a holistic entrepreneur, but these ancient healing methods certainly keep me on an even keel when I apply them.

Part I: Setting the Foundation

Chapter 1
Healthy Habits for
Vibrant Energy

E very day, in every moment, our cells are regenerating. The question is, how do you want your cells to regenerate? And what kind of energy do you want to go into those cells?

Cells are like sponges soaking up all that you feed them:

- Thoughts

- Food

- Experiences

- Chemical Gases

In this chapter, I'm going to share with you some lifestyle habits that are natural, mostly based on ancient practices and wisdom that will help you have more vibrancy in your life. These habits will set the foundation for my Vibrant Energy Flow System™ which I'll discuss in Chapter 2.

Holistic Healthy Habits

"Don't Be Caught with the Wrong Thoughts"

We all have to start somewhere. I say you start with the mind. The mind is a beautiful thing. It's like a computer. We program it to what we want it to think whether that be conscious or unconscious. Yep, what shows up in our life is what we have been thinking, and when we don't know how something showed up in our life, we have to understand that either something greater is guiding us or perhaps it is part of the 80 percent that we are unconscious about. You see, we are only about 20 percent conscious, and truthfully, the average person accesses only about 2 percent of her conscious thoughts.

The world has a set belief that as we age, our bodies start to breakdown. Aches and pain start to set in. Health challenges that our parents might have encountered are passed down to us. We are getting better at overcoming many types of cancer. We are concerned about what statistics show about the different decades of the aging process.

You can choose to buy into what the world's conscious beliefs are about aging. Or you can choose to have your own thoughts about aging. I have chosen to have the latter. Let me tell you that I have had a lot of beliefs to overcome since much of what I do today, I wasn't

encouraged to do as a young child. I'd never been encouraged to exercise and I wasn't taught to spend time in nature. I have chosen to
live my life very differently than what I grew up with.

So now it's time to ask you...If I were to wave a magic wand...

- What would you want your body to look like?
- How would you like your body to move?
- What kind of health would you like your body to have?

When women age, one of their biggest concerns is menopause.
Everyone thinks that you are "supposed" to have hot flashes and night
sweats, no sleep, and serious weight gain. This is a myth. We have
to be cognizant of what we are feeding our mind and what the people
around us are feeding it. Some of us are like sponges, soaking up all
the thoughts and things people are saying. I remember when one of
my family members was going through menopause. She had severe
hot flashes, and she projected all of her experiences onto her younger
family members who were right behind her in age, including myself.
However, I chose to cancel, delete, and reprogram my mind to know
that menopause could be the best years of my life.

I will admit that I went through a short phase of experiencing menopausal symptoms in my own life, but I chose to nip them in the bud by looking at what was truly causing them and applying the techniques described in this book.

I recently had one of my dance class friends comment on two pictures of me - one taken of me in my thirties and one of me now in my fifties. She said, "The pictures say that you can look great in your thirties, but you can look even better in your fifties." Truthfully, I feel like the picture in my thirties shows me concealing all the emotional and physical pain that I was dealing with back then, and my fifty something photo shows how vibrant I now feel.

What's happening on the inside can show up on the outside. It might not be apparent at first glance, but if someone were to look deeply, they can feel and see what's going on the inside. Emotions and thoughts do show up on the surface...so it's important to get your thoughts in alignment with how you want to experience life. Your thoughts will be the basis of how you move forward in embodying self-care rituals that can help you have vibrant health no matter what age you are. The goal is to be better than you were when you didn't have the experience and the wisdom that you now have in your mature years.

On that note, I would like for you to jot down some answers to the "magic wand" questions listed above so you can get started on setting the FOUNDATION for your journey to 30 Days to a Vibrant, Healthier, Younger You.

"Don't be Lenient with Convenience!"

Food is medicine. What you put into your body becomes you, based on the nutrients and the energy of the preparation.

Fast, take-out, pre-cooked and packaged food might be convenient for you at the time, but in the long run, is it the best choice for your body? All of these types of foods may well be prepared with high levels of sodium leaving you wondering why you have high blood pressure. And if you are already stressed, they will only add insult to your body's internal health challenges. It might seem overwhelming and burdensome but preparing your own meals will be one of the healthiest choices you can make for yourself and loved ones. If you don't have the convenience of working from home or a personal chef to prepare healthy holistic meals for you, take one day a week (Sunday, perhaps) to do meal prep for the entire week. Preparing meals can be very therapeutic.

Always use healthy, sustainable sources of food, whether you are a vegetarian, vegan, or an omnivore like me:

Animal Protein:

- Beef - organic and grass-fed (non-gmo)
- Chicken - organic and free range
- Fish and Shellfish - wild (not farm raised)
- Lamb - organic and grass-fed
- Pork - organic and grass-fed
- Turkey - organic and free range

Fruit: always organic (gmo-free)

Vegetables: always organic (gmo-free)

Best Ways to Cook/Prepare Your Food:

- Raw (during the warmer months and seasons)

- Steamed

- Baked

- Lightly broiled

- Lightly grilled

- Boiled

- Sauteed with water (only use oil for flavor after the food is cooked)

- With LOVE, always; when anger is in our cooking, it is passed on to the people eating the food and may show up as stomach aches, digestive issues, etc.

Notice that I didn't mention the microwave! The microwave is a modern convention that takes all the nutrients out of your food. If you wouldn't use it to heat your baby's milk, then guess what... it's not good for you either! If you have a microwave, you can use it to clean your sponges because it will kill all of the bacteria in them.

Oils that May be Used for Cooking:

- Avocado oil

- Ghee

- Coconut oil

- Grapeseed oil

Notice that I didn't list olive or flax oil. Olive oil and flax oil should not be heated; they should only be used for salad dressings or drizzled on cooked food.

Stay away from:
- Refined sugar (even if it's organic!)
- White flour
- Gluten (especially if you face health challenges with skin, lungs, allergies, autoimmune labels such lupus or multiple sclerosis, or mental health challenges such as ADD, ADHD, autism, bipolar disorder, or schizophrenia)
- Alcohol (use only occasionally to celebrate, not to drown your sorrows or de-stress)
- Coffee and other caffeinated drinks (they give you a false sense of energy)
- Nightshades (including tomatoes, eggplant, and peppers), especially if you have joint issues, autoimmune diseases, or any signs of inflammation in the body

All shelled nuts and seeds should be cleaned with grapefruit seed extract (GSE) solution, rinsed and soaked 24 hours in water before consuming. Because there can be enzyme inhibitors in nuts and seeds, soaking your nuts and seeds helps you to digest them easily.

It's always better if you use fresh seasonings with your food instead of dried seasonings; we don't know if the dried seasonings have mold or harmful bacteria from drying out. Grow an herb garden of:

- Sage
- Rosemary
- Thyme
- Basil
- Mint
- Oregano
- Marjoram

Our bodies also don't get enough minerals to keep it healthy. Here are some good sources of minerals:

- Himalayan or Sea Salt
- Seaweed (including dulse, kelp, or wakame) - Seaweed is

always great to season or cook with or eat as a snack.

- Green leafy vegetables - Eat as many possible cooked or raw:
  - Collards
  - Kale
  - Swiss chard
  - Mustard greens
  - Spinach
  - Romaine lettuce
  - Dandelion greens

The more color in your food, the more vibrancy it creates in your body and your life!

If you have digestive issues (e.g. bloating, flatulence, belching, etc.) then you definitely need to follow macrobiotic guidelines on food combining (for more information, see the article "Why Food Combining is Important?" at http://selfcarequeendom.com/self-care/macrobiotic/):

- Eat animal protein only with green leafy vegetables.
- Eat green leafy vegetables with animal protein or starchy

vegetables like carrots.

- If you are going to consume potatoes, then only eat red potatoes which have a low glycemic index.
- Fruit is always eaten by itself at least twenty minutes before consuming anything else.
- Melon should only be eaten alone at least an hour before consuming anything else.
- Grains, legumes, and beans can be consumed only with vegetables, whether they are green leafy vegetables or starchy.
- The only beverage to consume with meals is either hot tea or wine because anything else will dilute your own natural digestive enzymes needed to digest your food.

Fruit juice is nothing more than sugar, even if it is not refined. If you are trying to lose weight, do not drink fruit juice at all. The whole fruit is better off being eaten because it has fiber to help you eliminate easily and effortlessly.

"Stop Rockin' with the Toxins!"

Eliminate as many toxins as you can in your life! I am starting with a smoke-free, non-alcohol (or occasional drink for celebrations) lifestyle. Smoking ages you fast! Alcohol is fermented sugar, and sugar will age your skin quickly and affect your liver as well. I watched my dad die at the age of 67 after suffering from pancreatic cancer. He smoked and drank heavily when I was growing up, and my experience of him reflected what he was consuming; he was belligerent and prone to fits of rage. You think the toxicity from his liver having to process the alcohol had something to do with it?

Now when I talk about toxins, I'm talking about personal care products and household cleaning products as well. There are so many toxins in non-green, everyday cleaning products that we may be able to solve some of our chronic health challenges (e.g. coughing, wheezing and skin problems) if we just eliminated these toxins. There is less work for the body when it doesn't have to figure out what to do with the toxins that enter it. Honestly, the body reacts like a computer that hasn't been programmed to handle the toxins.

As a rule of thumb, if you can't pronounce the ingredients in a product then you probably shouldn't be using it on your body. For starters, you want to make sure all of your personal care products are free of parabens and sodium lauryl sulfate. These contaminants, which have been linked to causing cancer, disrupting the endocrine system, putting your hormones out of balance, and reproductive toxicity, can be disguised in your personal care products many ways. To get more information about this and a complete list of chemicals that you want to avoid in your personal care products, check out: http://www.safecosmetics.org/ .

Regarding your household cleaning products, you most definitely want to avoid bleach and ammonia, and ultimately the mixture of these two products, as they can create a chemical reaction of a cloud of gases that can damage your lungs. And avoid those sweet smelling fragrances in your laundry detergent, which may leave you with a headache, respiratory problems, sneezing, watery eyes and more. I remember staying at a friend's house and when I walked in her home, I could immediately smell the chemicals from the laundry. My head not only hurt, but my eyes were red and watery. My first guess was that her laundry detergent didn't gel with me as I'm used to avoiding irritants and chemicals in such products.

The best solution is to create your own cleaning products, and you will find that many of your allergies and health projects begin to improve.

Ingredients needed to create cleaning products:

- Dr. Bronner's Castile Soap
- Peppermint, lemon, orange essential oils
- Olive oil to help clean wood surfaces
- Distilled water
- Baking soda (if you want some scrubbing power)
- Hydrogen peroxide

On a larger level, if you own your home, you might want to consider hardwood floors and tile instead of carpet. New carpet has Volatile Organic Compounds (VOCs) which include highly toxic chemicals such as formaldehyde and acetaldehyde, along with benzene, toluene, perchloroethylene, and more. (Can you pronounce all of those words?) In the short term, such as immediately after new carpeting is installed, VOCs may cause health challenges such as headaches, nausea, and nerve problems, along with irritation to your eyes, nose, and throat. Plus, if you have chronic asthma or allergies, you might notice that they improve or disappear without the carpet.

I noticed that when I moved to a home with hardwood floors, my long-standing breathing challenges disappeared completely.

Also, when you paint, use no-VOC paint, because the toxins can cause all kinds of health challenges as mentioned above with the carpet. I can speak volumes on this as a holistic practitioner who painted my session rooms using no-VOC paint. I remember my nephew helped me paint one of my offices, and he told me that I didn't need to go to such extremes and buy expensive paint. I remember telling him that I help people with their health challenges, so I'm not going to create more health challenges for them by creating a toxic environment for them to receive sessions. Later, my nephew finished the job for me and was amazed how there were no toxic fumes and how much better he felt doing the job. He endorsed my choice of no-VOC paint after his experience of painting my session room.

Get started by getting rid of all the toxins in your household that may be keeping you sick with chronic health challenges. I have to tell you that when I cleaned this area up in my life, my breathing challenges went away. Where can you start? Start small, perhaps with just your makeup and skincare. Regarding skincare, using just pure oil on your skin is better than lotion. Here's what my skincare friend Erin Massengale of Danu Skincare shared with me many years ago-- "When we make lotion and add water, we have to put in a preservative so it doesn't oxidize and go bad. It is best to just use an oil such as avocado oil when you get out of the shower or bathtub." That's your lotion: oil on wet skin. It's actually less expensive to buy yourself a large bottle of avocado oil (it helps create supple skin, which is important when you are over 40!) and slather it over your body when you get out of the shower.

Be Wise with the Exercise!

Exercising on a daily basis is great, but I recommend that you do something that feeds your soul. For example, I love to dance, so I take dance classes twice a week. The little girl inside of me (my inner child) gets to have fun with the dance movements as my adult body enjoys the cardio workout that it gives my heart and body. Another way I work out and feed my soul is hiking in nature. I love communing with nature as a daily spiritual practice. It's a way to clear my mind and to connect with Spirit. Unbeknownst to me at the time, I had been hiking 2.1 miles daily, on average, while communing with nature. I shed pounds without even trying, and my core seemed to be stronger. It worked for me because I am not the type of girl who goes to the gym to do squats and lift weights...that's just not my cup of tea. Instead, I strengthened my core during warm ups in dance and increased my stamina through hiking.

I have a friend and client, Ruby, who loves to go for daily walks to feed the kitties in her neighborhood. I remember her telling me that she could never get down to a size 4. After watching her for a year or so, doing some of the daily ancient rituals presented in this book plus exercising naturally, her body went from a size 14 to a size 4. She was amazed by the results!

A senior client of mine enjoys swimming and swims 5 days a week in the morning. I leave you with this question: What activity do you like to engage in that gives your body movement and feeds your soul (and yes, sex can count...but it's not the only activity to engage in)?

The Missing Link to Vibrant Health

Some people go get acupuncture, chiropractic adjustments or other modalities done on themselves once or twice a week. I think these are great treatments when you have a long withstanding problem that needs to be handled. The key is: How do you maintain your body daily by yourself?

You have tools right at your fingertips to help you on a daily basis and even at a moment's notice. Every day, when we wake up, we step into a vortex of the world and all of its energies. Sometimes we are blindsided by what we are hit with; other times, we can feel it coming on. Many of us are empathic and don't know what energies we are feeling, so we wonder what is wrong with us. The cleaner we keep our energy, the less likely we are to take on someone else's energies. After my introduction to the Asian Healing Arts in 1996 while experiencing extreme fatigue and a compromised immune system, I decided to delve deeper to learn more about what exactly this type of healing was and why it worked. It quickly became a part of my daily regimen, and I knew that I had to go study acupressure/ Chinese Medicine, Jin Shin Jyutsu and Shamanic work. Eventually in 2011 the Vibrant Energy Flow System™ was born!

The Vibrant Energy Flow System™ is a blend of the most potent material from acupressure, a Japanese healing art called Jin Shin Jyutsu, and the Chakra Balancing System. My originally released audio version of the Vibrant Energy Flow System™ included quick, daily Self-Care Rituals to help keep you balanced and solve health challenges in ways that might leave your physicians scratching their heads, wondering why it worked instead of medication. It is the very thing that stopped all of my frantic, mommy-wearing trips to the pediatrician's office to figure out what was wrong with my daughters. I even had my pediatrician ask how I kept my daughters so healthy because she only saw them for well-care visits. I remember revealing in a secretive, matter-of-fact way that I was a healing arts practitioner and therefore kept my girls healthy with good nutrition and my hands-on healing. The pediatrician was very supportive and said to me, "I think it's great! Whatever works!"

To put it simply, we human beings have electromagnetic fields, just like our electronic devices. We are quite sensitive when our energy fields start leaking energy or experiencing tears. An argument or conflict can cause such an energy leakage or tears. Sometimes we are very giving individuals (rescuers, I like to call us, always ready to help others), and we wonder why we suddenly feel tired when we are around certain individuals. Well, others feel our energy and want to take it from us, so they do. We are vulnerable and don't know what's hit us, when really, on the energetic level, someone has taken our energy. Many walk around feeling depleted all the time, and some go get help from an energy healer like myself. Illnesses such as an everyday cold or flu or serious life threatening illnesses can cause our inner circuitry to go haywire. Therefore, the Vibrant Energy Flow System™ can help rewire our inner energetic circuitry. When we rewire our inner circuitry, we can relax, recharge, and restore our energy, resulting in us feeling vibrant and looking youthful.

Some may think that I am pulling this information out of a hat, but what I am sharing is an integration of healing modalities that have been around for more than 5000 years, long before Western medicine was even born. Many esteemed doctors, including Andrew Weil, MD, who is known for his integrative and holistic approach to medicine, endorse touch therapies similar to the Vibrant Energy Flow System™ - "Because there is such a profound connection between mind and body, anything that can put a person in a state of relaxation can be a great benefit. Studies have shown that when a person is deeply relaxed, heart rate and blood pressure decrease, blood flow to the bowels and bladder increases and breathing becomes rhythmic and slow. This creates an optimal environment for the body's natural immune resources to take over and promote healing." (http://www.drweil.com/health-wellness/balanced-living/wellness-therapies/healing-touch/)

Christiane Northrup, MD, an OBGYN who believes in the integrative approach to medicine, states in the forward of Donna Eden's book, *Energy Medicine for Women* - "I began experimenting with energy medicine in my gynecological practice many years ago, using it when I had to perform invasive office procedures such as endometrial biopsies, the removal of IUDs,or tests that involved ejection of the dye into the uterus. I sensed how disruptive these routine procedures were to the body's natural energy fields, so as the final part of the treatment, I would have my patient lie down and I would move my hands in long passes above her body. Something in this simple act seemed to help restabilize the body's energy fields. Many women would report immediate relief of pain or cramps, pleasurable tingling sensations in the areas that had been traumatized or deepening calm throughout their bodies...Your hands hold powerful medicine - "energy medicine" - that beyond just soothing the body after an invasive procedure is able to prevent or help overcome challenging illnesses."

With all this talk about the credibility of hands-on healing, let's get you started with the Vibrant Energy Flow System™.

Chapter 2
The Vibrant Energy Flow System™

The Vibrant Energy Flow System™ is a blend of the most potent parts of a few ancient healing modalities including Chinese Medicine and the seven energy centers called the Chakra Healing System, which dates back to more than 5000 years. These energy flow techniques will help you rewire your inner circuitry, thus sustaining your health and wellbeing in all aspects: mind, body and spirit. Many find that emotionally charged issues diminish the more they apply this system to their bodies and bio-energetic fields. Other benefits of the Vibrant Energy Flow System™ include deep relaxation, diminished pain, and I even had one of my yogi clients say, "Feeling like you are plugged into Source!"

I've spent the past 19 years giving thousands of sessions to men and women to help them find vibrant energy in their lives, ranging from maintaining their bodies during daily stresses to the extreme of combatting serious life threatening diseases such as cancer. Now, I'm going to be honest--not everyone who had cancer survived it--but those who did were consistently receiving this work in conjunction with traditionally Western medicine treatments. When the Vibrant Energy Flow System is practiced as a daily ritual, my clients usually report that their day goes much smoother, and they feel energized in a peacefully calm way.

In this particular book, I will introduce 5 energy patterns to you to get you started along with a few quick release holds to help you with everyday or seasonal health related issues. Using these flow patterns will bring you increased vibrant energy and health to support you in your work and personal life. I'm inviting you to give yourself 20 to 30 minutes a day to practice self care so that you can be a clear channel for yourself and your people (family, friends and/or clients).

Guidelines for Practicing Flow Patterns

1) Lie down on your back/side or sit in a chair, thus allowing gravity to support you.

2) Use your palms, back of your hand, and fingers (but not your thumbs!). We'll focus on techniques that avoid creating stress and strain on the body.

3) As we work through each flow pattern, breathwork is purposefully included. The breathwork will help you re-

lease and let go of any armor preventing anything other than light and love. Consider this breathwork to be a meditative practice.

These flow patterns can be used everywhere--before climbing out of bed or before going to sleep, in the middle of the day, or even when sitting in a chair. Heck, I even use them while I am sungazing.

You might find your body relaxing in ways you've never imagined. There will be energetic releases that may take the form of:

- Gurgling from your abdominal cavity
- Twitching muscles
- Heat being released from the body
- Unexpected sounds coming from your mouth such as sighing
- Changes in breathing patterns

...And yes, bodily gases may be released as well. Understand that this is just your body's way of unleashing unbalanced energies.

Chapter 3
How to Stay the Course and Be Wildly Successful with the Vibrant Energy Flow System™

The Vibrant Energy Flow System™ is an energy healing modality that detoxifies your body. Warning: If you have been neglecting your body, you could go through some serious jolts of healing. I don't say this to scare you, but I want you to be aware that your body will be going through a metamorphosis if it isn't used to feeling clean energetically.

At one point in my own healing, I stopped doing the Vibrant Energy Flow System™ on myself and went to get an intense series of sessions of one of the modalities embedded in the Vibrant Energy Flow System™. When I came home, my left hip was in excruciating pain. It was an interesting dilemma because here I was a practitioner of ten years and my body was screaming with pain, but what I realized was that what was showing up as hip pain was really my body crying with emotions. You see, not only had we just lost three family members within 45 days, but my husband at the time had recently quit his job without working out with me first how we were going to make ends meet without draining our savings. So I embodied all kinds of emotions that left me sad, angry, and frustrated, and this manifested as pain in my left hip. Note: the left side of the body is all about emotions. Hip pain can come from frustration.

After I got home from these intense sessions, I also had my mentor at the time work on me, using acupuncture needles. Let's just say that I was still in pain and DESPERATE. You know that you are in a lot of pain when you can't stand needles, but you will let an acupuncturist put them in you to do whatever it takes to relieve the pain.

Even after all of this, I felt like I needed more help. I remember limping to one of my offices and trying to get another acupuncturist there to treat me. Our schedules clashed so that wasn't going to work. Guess what? I had no choice but to resort to my own hands. I began to re-acquaint myself with the self-contained flow patterns and performed them on myself on a daily basis. After about 20 days or so, I started to notice that the pain was gone. I remember telling someone the story about how I was in so much pain initially after my intense sessions but that now my left hip pain was gone. So what I am conveying here is that sometimes things will get worse before they get better; so it's important to stick with the flow patterns and be disciplined about it. Build them into your life as self-care rituals and pretty soon you will find that the pain will diminish.

I want to share another story with you about a business friend of mine who had an asthma challenge. She mentioned to me that she was better since she had lowered her consumption of alcohol and dealt with her emotions instead. She told me that her doctor had diagnosed her with asthma. I mentioned to her, "You know that I pretty much healed myself from asthma, right?"

Before I finish this story, I want to tell you as a practitioner of almost 20 years, that asthma is not the same for each individual who encounters it. Secondly, I would prefer to call it a "breathing" project. When you give it the label asthma, then it owns you and you embody it. When you say a breathing project then it means you are working on a project concerning your breath and exploring ways to complete your goal of breathing better. Let's define project - an individual or collaborative enterprise that is carefully planned and designed to achieve a particular aim. A breathing project is aimed at helping you stop having breathing difficulties.

Anyhow, I quickly assessed my friend's breathing project and realized that a flow incorporating the LIVER meridian would prove most helpful to her. She came back after doing the RELIEVE THE STRESS flow pattern (included in the soon to be released Vibrant Energy Flow System™ 2.0) on herself and told me that she felt like she was coming down with a cold. She then began to share with me how she has had really bad seasonal allergies in the past. I immediately shared with her that the same flow pattern helps with bad allergies as well and to continue doing it even it feels like she's coming down with something.

So you see, your body might go through a detox while doing the Vibrant Energy Flow System™. If that happens, you are going to want to go back to your old habits. You will unconsciously want to sway the way that is most familiar and comfortable for you. But don't. During detox, it's more important than ever to pull from all of your health and wellness tools and stay on the train. Continue doing the flows. Make sure you drink lots of water and are prioritizing eating cleanly. If you find that doing the flows is a little too much for you, seek support in my Vibrant Energy Flow System™ Facebook

Group, where you will meet several people who have been utilizing the flows and me popping in to answer your questions. You might want to enroll yourself in the forthcoming Vibrant Energy Flow System™ 2.0 Home Study Program to get more support and exposure to flows that may help you move through the detoxing symptoms that are coming up for healing.

However, I want to stress how important it is to rest and listen to your body and notice if you are feeling like you want to go grab a piece of candy or have a glass of wine or a salty snack. This is the time to pay attention to what flow is going to help you diminish a particular craving and dissolve the emotions around what you are feeling. The Vibrant Energy Flow System™ is designed to help you on all levels, mentally, emotionally and physically, thus touching into the depths of your soul.

You might want to earmark this chapter, so that when you get stuck on a particular day, you can come back and remind yourself to stay on the train of health and wellness.

Part II:
The 30 Day Challenge to Get into Action

Chapter 1: Day 1
Exhaling to Allow the Abundance In

Breathwork is such an important component of this work. When breathing and doing the Vibrant Energy Flows it is important to exhale first. Exhaling is about letting go, and inhaling is about receiving. So many people walk around with shallow breath, they are holding their breath. Often, people tell you to inhale first. However, I always start with exhaling. Exhaling allows you to let go; it allows you to release dead air that has been trapped inside of you and just sits there because you haven't finished exhaling. When you don't allow yourself to complete your exhalation, you cannot fully receive with the next breath. So in order to inhale, you must fully exhale. This is a true metaphor for anything in our lives. In order to receive, we must let go of old situations in our lives that don't work in order to receive abundantly. Before you do anything in this book, you need to learn how to breathe deeply. The Vibrant Energy Flow System™ naturally helps you to breathe deeply; thus, it is a great meditative activity helping you to receive abundantly. In this first chapter, we are laying the groundwork to learn how to breathe deeply. Right now, take this moment to exhale first and then inhale.

Do it about eight more times, noticing that as you exhale more and let go, how deeply you are able to inhale, thus receiving the breath of LIFE. Take note of how cleansing it may feel for you.

Chapter 2: Day 2
Center Yourself So
You May Receive

Most of us are comfortable giving, but when it comes to receiving…some of us are a little uncomfortable.

So we start by sitting or lying down. Yes, it can be done standing up, but it's not recommended as the flow pattern will take about 15 to 20 minutes to complete.

CENTERING FLOW

Step 1: Put your right hand on top of the crown of your head, and place

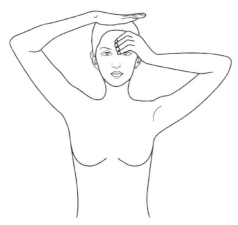 your left fingers between your eyebrows (known as the Third Eye). Breathe for about 3-4 breath cycles; exhaling first, then inhaling is one breath cycle. Exhaling first allows you to LET GO, so you may receive when you INHALE.

Step 2: Keep your right hand on the crown of your head, while moving your left fingers to the tip of your nose. Again, breathe 3-4 four breath cycles... exhaling first, then inhaling.

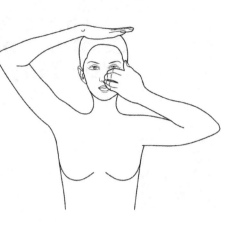

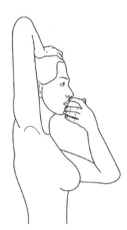

Step 3: Next, place your left index finger in the small, center, hollow space between your nose and upper lip (called the philtrum) and the left middle and ring fingers in the center indentation just below your lower lip and chin. Breathe 3-4 breath cycles...exhaling first then inhaling.

Step 4: Move your left fingers to the center hollow area between the neck and just above the collar (clavicle) bone, where the throat meets the clavicle. Again, breathe 3-4 breath cycles.

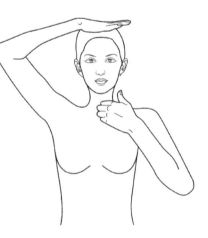

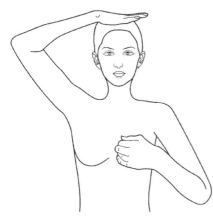

Step 5: Now move left fingers to the center indentation between the breast bones. Breathe 3-4 breath cycles.

Step 6: Place the left fingers at the base of the sternum where the left and right ribs meet the sternum (xiphoid process). (Note: Be careful not to press here. It may be best to palm the area so that you don't knock the wind out of yourself.)

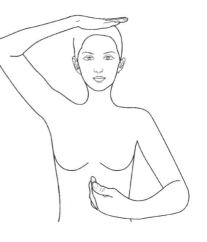

Breathe 3-4 breath cycles.

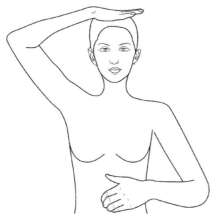

Step 7: Place your left fingers just above the belly button, and breathe 3-4 breath cycles.

Step 8: Next, palm your pubic bone, and breathe 3-4 breath cycles.

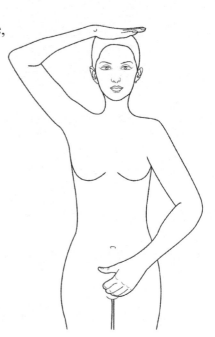

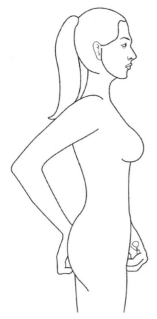

Step 9: Finally, move your right hand to your tailbone (known as the coccyx) while your left hand stays put. Breathe 3-4 breath cycles.

Notice how you feel. Do you feel centered? Grounded? If you were feeling hormonal before, you might sense a feeling of emotional release. Yes, the Centering Flow can affect your hormones in a great way; each of the areas that your left hand navigated down on the core of your body were connected to the endocrine system (the physiological name for your hormonal system).

Hence, this Centering Flow is a wonderful flow to do at night just before falling asleep to help you with any sleep disorders such as insomnia. It can also help you with your memory and affect the immune system in a positive way so that you don't get as many colds or flus. If you are pre-diabetic or even diabetic, this flow can help you balance your blood sugar levels. Last but not least, if you often find yourself tired and reaching for caffeine at 3 in the afternoon, you might find this flow helps you to have more energy.

For those with thyroid projects such as Graves or even Hashimoto's disease, the Centering Flow could improve your thyroid. It also balances the pH level of your blood so that you aren't leaching calcium from your bones, which causes osteoporosis.

Besides helping the hormones, the Centering Flow is a great overall flow to do on yourself to help you get ready for your day and any life challenges that might be thrown at you. Better yet, it promotes peaceful slumber at the end of the day, clearing you of energies faced earlier on that might have challenged you mentally, emotionally, or even physically.

Chapter 3: Day 3
The Preventative Flow
for the Common Cold or Flu
(Attitude Adjustment Flow)

S imple but yet powerful, the Attitude Adjustment Flow helps you to shift the state of your being. What exactly does this mean? Suppose you are worrying a lot, and you have what the Buddhist call a "monkey mind" that just won't shut off. Much of our attitudes or emotions have a lot to do with our inability to control a situation, so instead of going with the flow (which the Attitude Adjustment Flow will help you shift into), you allow your "monkey mind," fear, or even raging hormones to overtake you. You end up projecting all of your "stuff" onto people or situations you come in contact with, whether that be the car that you are driving next to, your children and their lives, or even fear about living in today's world with all the terrorism going on.

Metaphysically speaking, a cold or flu usually has to do with mental and emotional congestion. So, if you are harboring all of these negative thoughts or feelings, then you are setting yourself up for a weakened immune system, thus making yourself vulnerable to a cold or flu. We all have been there. Before I talk about this flow, I want to share a story about a long-term client of mine.

I had a client who had nearly freaked out at the whole anthrax scare right after 9/11. This client went and purchased equipment and food in anticipation of a crisis. My empathic skills sensed FEAR all over this client. Every time this client came for a session, I would always hear the causal level of FEAR in my assessment tools. Thus, I worked on this client from the perspective of FEAR. This client also had frequent colds. Eventually, after working on shifting beliefs and thought patterns, my client stopped catching colds as often, AND I stopped hearing this person project the same FEAR about anthrax or other possible terrorist attacks.

To get started, choose a side that you want to work on as this flow is bilateral (which means that you can do it on either side or on both separately). Note that the left side is usually the emotional side and generational beliefs and consciousness, and the right side is usually connected more to lifestyle habits.

Step 1: Put your opposite hand on the opposite shoulder. For example, right hand goes on the left shoulder for the left flow and vice versa for the right flow. Make sure that the palm of your hand is on the top of the shoulders and your fingers fall between the top edge of the shoulder blade and the spine. Put your knees together (it is easiest to do this while lying on your side). Now make a ring with your thumb and index finger (Note: the thumb pad should be touching the fingernail of the index finger). Breathe about 9 breath cycles for each finger.

Right Flow   **Left Flow**

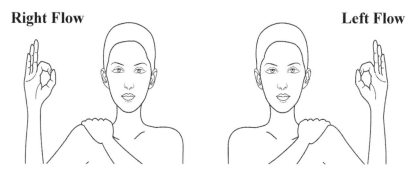

Step 2: Then bring the thumb pad to the middle fingernail...9 breath cycles.

Right Flow   **Left Flow**

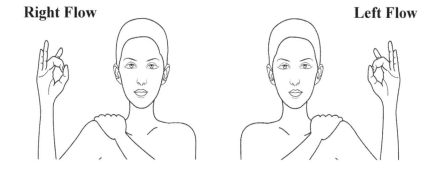

Step 3: Thumb pad to ring fingernail…9 breath cycles.

Right Flow   **Left Flow**

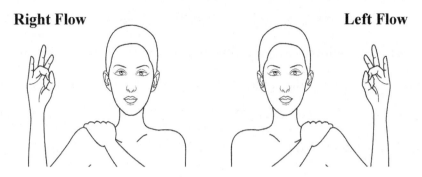

Step 4: Thumb pad to baby fingernail…9 breath cycles.

Right Flow   **Left Flow**

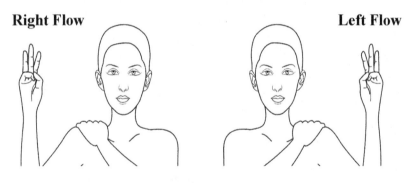

Switch sides with opposite shoulder and repeat the steps above for the side that you didn't complete.

Remember to BREATHE!

As you do this flow, you will be helping yourself shift or diminish an attitude or emotion; the thumb is about worry; the index finger is about fear; the middle finger is about anger; the ring finger is about sadness and grief; and the baby finger is about perfection and feeling overwhelmed. Ultimately, you are helping or starting the process of letting go of all of your baggage! I say in process because the more you do this, the more you let go on a different and deeper layer.

With bilateral flows, the left side is usually emotional and the right side is about shifting the lifestyle habits. Understand that the left side of the body also includes generational pieces that you may be unconscious about...and this could include attitudes, beliefs and behaviors passed down from your ancestral lineage.

Chapter 4: Day 4
The Vibrant Energy Flow System™ as a Daily Ritual

Incorporating the Vibrant Energy Flow System™ daily into your life is a special gift that you can give to yourself. Some people may meditate daily, some people spend time in nature, and some people do yoga poses first thing in the morning. You can integrate this work with your meditation practice or even on your hikes and definitely with yoga poses.

One of my business healing clients shared this with me in 2011 after taking one of my self hands-on healing classes: "I went out for a walk in the late evening in my neighborhood. I noticed that it was starting to get dark. I am not a runner, but I felt like I needed to sprint back home before it got dark since I was out all alone. I started running, and then I remembered one of the hand poses that you taught us in class. So I did it! I made a ring with my thumb pad and ring fingernail on both sides, and when I got home I felt like a racehorse ready for a race."

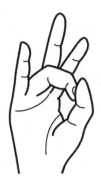 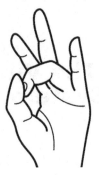

Truthfully, I myself am almost always multi-processing when I do the Vibrant Energy Flow System™. Often I go for a morning hike, and on that hike, I stop and do my daily practice of sungazing. While sungazing you can often find me doing hand poses and breathing, and even when I am done with the hand poses and still have time left to sungaze, I will actually start doing the Attitude Adjustment Flow.

I believe I shared in one of the earlier chapters that one of my healing colleagues and yogi clients described the Vibrant Energy Flow System™ as a way of plugging into Source/Spirit. Well, we can also say that meditation is a way to plug into Source/Spirit, right? Many do meditation to quiet their mind. What if you could quiet your mind quicker by doing the Vibrant Energy Flow System™?

To me, doing the Vibrant Energy Flow System™ is a meditative practice in itself. It will allow you to focus on your breath and quiet the chatter going on in your head...or clear it out for that matter so that you remember who you are on a soul level.

The five flows included in this book can all be done within an hour, or one of them can easily be done in 20 minutes or less. You can also do any combination of the flows that you feel called to do, given what they can help you with.

Some days, I do all five flows, and other days I do only hand poses or just one flow. Or maybe, I'll do one in the morning and one at night. Some of my clients have reported doing a few of the flows in the morning and one or two at night before going into a deep slumber. Whatever you choose, I say try it out, and see what works for you. The key is to get you to a place of accessing these flows from memory so when you do need them, you know exactly what to do.

The Vibrant Energy Flow System™ can be used alone or with other movement modalities or practices. If you are already meditating daily, you might want to experience one of the Vibrant Energy Flows that you have learned thus far while meditating. The one I would suggest is the Attitude Adjustment Flow (See Appendix – Illustration 2), or you may use the hand pose that gives you stamina that I mentioned earlier in this chapter.

Chapter 5: Day 5
Energizing Sunshine for the Body

The morning sun is my favorite. When I go for a morning hike, it's actually fun to sungaze and feel Father Sun not only warming up my body but providing energy for my body. As an alternative to the actual sun, the Energizing Flow is actually like bringing sunlight into your body, warming you up and energizing you with focused energy. Yep, you read that right; the Energizing Flow is like putting sunshine in your body! On those mornings when the sun is hiding behind the cloud cover (thus preventing me from sungazing), this is my go-to flow. As a matter of fact, it was my go-to flow long before I started sungazing. This flow is for you if you don't have the discipline to go outside right after the sun rises or sets to sungaze daily or if you want your energy to be focused and less scattered. Much like we get Vitamin D from the sun, this flow will also help strengthen your immune system because it helps the biggest lymph node in your system, the spleen. In Chinese Medicine, part of learning and memorizing facts comes from having the spleen energy in balance so that is why the Energizing Flow actually helps you have more focused energy as well. I highly recommend doing this flow daily if you are a person who seems to always be running on "empty." It is one of the best flows to help you with fatigue that I share in this book and my DVD product - *30 Days to a Vibrant, Healthier, Younger You* (http://www.selfcarequeendom.com/30days).

The Energizing Flow is bilateral - meaning that it has a right flow and a left flow. You don't have to do both flows daily. Choosing one side to do daily is good enough to ensure that you have focused energy. Will it be helpful if you do both sides? You bet it would; however, it isn't necessary. You can choose which side you would like to do daily based on how you might be feeling. Understand that left flows are usually helping emotional and ancestral pieces and the right flows generally help with lifestyle challenges. For example, if you are always a person who worries and it seems to be a behavior/attitude that runs in your family, then the left flow would be beneficial. The right flow would be a good one to do if you are always tired and craving or eating sweets and/or carbohydrates.

To get started with the Right Energizing Flow follow the diagram (also referenced in the Appendix as Illustration 3):

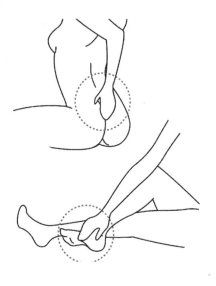

Step 1: First, put your right hand on the arch of your right foot and left palm on your tailbone. Breath 3-4 breath cycles.

Step 2: Place your right fingers a hand's-width up from your right inside ankle (left hand remains on the tailbone, also known as the coccyx). Breathe 3 or 4 breaths.

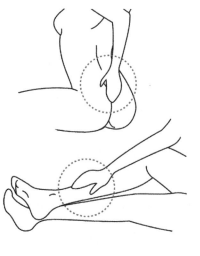

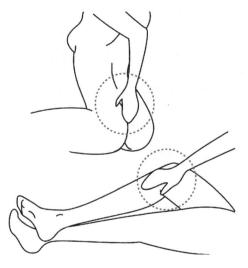

Step 3: Place your right fingers just below the inside of your right knee. Breathe 3 or 4 breaths.

Step 4: Next, place your right fingers in your right groin area. Breathe 3 or 4 breath cycles.

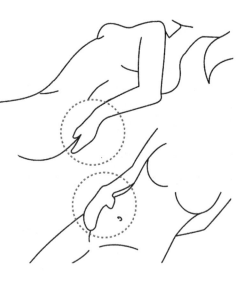

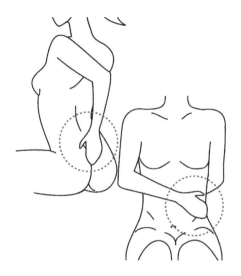

Step 5: Now, move your right hand to the base of your left, front ribs. Breathe 3 or 4 breath cycles.

Step 6: Place left hand a hand's-width down from the right clavicle, which is in vertical alignment with the right ear (when your head is facing forward). Breathe 3-4 more breath cycles.

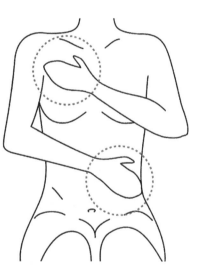

Step 7: Your left hand moves to the base of the left clavicle, in vertical alignment with the left ear when looking forward. Note that you can clean out the whole area underneath the clavicle (collar-bone) by coming close to the sternum, then out towards the shoulder joint ana-

tomically known as the glenohumeral joint.

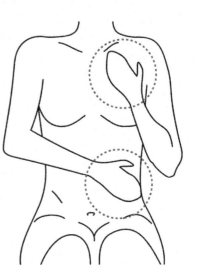

You can reverse the sides by exchanging the orientation of the sides with hands and sides of the body. See Illustration 3 for the Left flow in the Appendix.

If you would prefer an instructional video, you might want to purchase the online virtual product - *30 Days to a Vibrant, Healthier, Younger You* (http://www.selfcarequeendom.com/30days). This product will not only give you the instructional visual to do the flow pattern, but there's an audio MP3 download included to help guide you once you know how to find the areas on your body.

Chapter 6: Day 6
Oil Pulling, an Ancient Healing Method to Detox the Body

Oil pulling is a daily ritual borrowed from Ayurvedic Medicine. It is a healthy way to take care of your gums and pull the toxins out of your body while strengthening your immune system.

Yes, I have oil pulled and engaged in the Vibrant Energy Flow System™ at the same time. Here's the deal with oil pulling--it is done for 20 minutes and can be easily done while multi-tasking.

Here are the reasons why you want to oil pull:

Benefits of Oil pulling

★ Reduces bacteria in your system
    Healthier gums
    Stops tooth decay
    Prevents bad breath

★ *Pulls the toxins out of your system*
    Improve skin conditions - acne,
  eczema, psoriasis
    Healthier immune system
    Clears your sinuses

★ *Whitens your teeth (forget those teeth*
  whitening strips)

One day my tooth was hurting me, and I didn't want to go to the dentist to hear that I had a cavity to be filled, so I decided to try this whole oil pulling technique that I had heard about through one of my Facebook friends. Since then, I have been oil pulling daily since 2013. My teeth are white, my gums are healthy, and I didn't need to get a cavity filled.

I highly recommend this practice as a way to take care of your teeth and gums and to help you build a healthy immune system. Please note that you still need to floss daily, but this oil pulling business takes care of your teeth on a whole other level.

How to oil pull:

Take a teaspoon of unrefined oil, preferably coconut oil but oils such as sesame or olive oil can be used as well (if you are allergic to coconut oil or don't particularly like the taste or smell). Swish it around your mouth for about twenty minutes. Multitasking and doing other things around the house while oil pulling will help the time go by fast and make it easier to complete the entire 20 minutes.

Here are some guidelines to keep in mind when oil pulling -

- Please be sure that you do not swallow the oil. If you swallow, then it's like you're putting all the bad bacteria and toxins back into your system. (Note: You can get very sick if you swallow.) Oil pulling is best done on an empty stomach, which is why I recommend doing it first thing in the morning.

- You must swish around the mouth for about twenty minutes to get great coverage so you allow the bad bacteria to cling to the oil.

- When the twenty minutes are up, I highly suggest that you spit the oil in a plastic bag, not down your sink or in the toilet because it could clog your plumbing.

In addition to oil pulling, I recommend that you stop using all the commercial toothpastes on the market...even the ones that you buy at the health food stores. Here's the deal-- most toothpastes have vegetable glycerin. Glycerin is a sticky substance that coats the teeth while brushing thus setting your teeth up to attract more plaque. Plaque is a recipe for tooth decay and gum disease if not removed properly. Hence, I am recommending a tooth cleanser from Rupam Herbals that not only eliminates these ingredients, but has some great ingredients to fortify your teeth with minerals to nourish them so that you can avoid tooth decay as well as bone and gum loss (http://www. rupamherbalstore.com/one-drop-only/).

Chapter 7: Day 7
Boost Your Immunity
with Probiotics

After oil pulling first thing in the morning, you want to take a probiotic. You might already know what a probiotic is...if you don't know what a probiotic is, here's the explanation of what it is, why you need to take it, and how to take it.

Probiotics are healthy bacteria and yeast to aid your digestive system. Honestly the gut is full of both healthy and bad bacteria, so to combat the bad bacteria, we ingest probiotics. Probiotics are especially helpful after you have taken a course of antibiotics. As you may well know, antibiotics are great for fending off bad bacteria in the body, but unfortunately they fend off all bacteria, the good and the bad, stripping you of the good bacteria needed to properly digest your food and to balance the bad stuff that shows up from foods or infections we may have encountered from a cold or flu. Yep, probiotics are great for keeping a healthy immune system intact. Some research has shown that probiotics have been helpful in skin conditions such as eczema, fending off colds and flus, oral health, and keeping vaginal and bladder infections at bay. The best way to take probiotics is on an empty stomach so that you minimize stomach acids from killing off the live micro-organisms from the probiotics. When you put food in the mix, stomach acid is produced to break down food matter thus destroying the live organism of the probiotics.

Not all probiotics are equal and do the same thing. There are different probiotics for the stomach, the small intestine and the large intestine. Healthy Trinity by Natren covers the full spectrum from the stomach to the large intestine. I find that many people have taken heavy dosages of antibiotics but who haven't been on probiotics before would probably benefit from starting here. Later, if you know that you have issues with your large intestine or small intestine, such as diverticulitis or irritable bowel syndrome (which is mixture of constipation and loose stools), then you will want a probiotic specifically for your large intestine called *bifidum*. *Lactobacillus* is best for the small intestine and oral care.

After taking a probiotic, wait at least 30 minutes (preferably an hour) before eating.

Chapter 8: Day 8
Enzymatic Power!

Notice that I am slowly sprinkling in different practices to help you achieve or maintain your very own vibrancy. Vibrancy comes from within; it is not just about taking care of your body, but really loving yourself inside-out and WANTING to take care of yourself and your body, not because you have to but because you want to!

Today, I am going to introduce something to you if you don't already have it in your daily regimen. It is Enzymatic Power. As we age, our natural digestive enzymes diminish. Most of us dilute them when we drink with our meals. The only two beverages that can help promote digestion are hot tea and wine. These two beverages have natural enzymes in them to help warm up the digestive system so that you can digest your food with ease.

We need our digestive enzymes to obtain the proper nutrition from our food. One way to get digestive enzymes is to start your day with juicing raw vegetables. Notice I didn't include fruit. Wanna know why? Fruit is nothing more than sugar when you juice it.

When you turn fruit into sugar and consume it, you may be spiking and confusing your body with high blood sugar levels. Also, if you are a person who has issues with candida[1] you might find that you just exasperate your digestive system.

Here's a recipe for a green drink that I am passing onto you that I received from an orthomolecular nutritionist who helped me heal myself from a bleeding colon (after every Western doctor wanted to put me under the knife to remove it without thoroughly examining my case to see what was really going on):

Green Drink Recipe

- 5 leaves of romaine lettuce
- 4-5 celery stalks
- 1 small zucchini (or a big zucchini cut into smaller portions)
- Half of cucumber

Put in your juicer and drink up first thing in the morning before you put any other food into your system (after oil pulling and taking probiotics).

---

1   Candida is a parasitic fungi that can appear in the mouth (as thrush), intestinal tract or the vagina. It is often benign, but can become pathogenic and be the root of many health challenges.

Chapter 9: Day 9
Getting Unstuck in Body, Mind & Spirit

M ovement is good. Going with the flow is even great-er! Creating harmony in your life is imperative. Oftentimes, we get stuck in our minds, which in return shows up in our bodies. I hate to tell you this, but it does show up on your face as well. You know those worry lines we get on our faces, like we've been thinking too hard? When you get stuck in the same thoughts over and over again, worry lines may show up on your face. You have to pull yourself out of this vicious thinking cycle.

It is a feeling of being stuck in the mud about everything. Have you ever felt like you were stuck in mud? It's hard to move, and even your muscles feel like they can't really move...right? Many times that can happen after you've been stuck with a flu-bug for three weeks too long, and when you go to move your arms and legs, it takes everything in you to move because your limbs feel heavy with excess mucous in your tissues. It feels very taxing to even think about moving, right? So, here's a flow I've got for you to help you through those times of feeling stuck: the Anti-Aging Flow!

The Anti-Aging Flow is best used at night to help you clear your thoughts and energies from the day (See Illustration 4 in the Appendix).

The Anti-Aging Flow helps you with exactly what it is called, Anti-Aging. Truth be told, all of those "monkey mind" thoughts and frustrating repercussions from those thoughts show up on your face, whether you like it or not. I don't care how much skincare or make-up you use; they show up. The way to help relax those lines on your face is to apply the Anti-Aging Flow. I recommend doing it at night, but you can do it any time of the day. But doesn't it make sense to do this flow at night to help clear the mental activities of the day? The anchor point of this flow is all about helping you to escape from your very own mental bondage. Imagine the great sleep a person with a lot on their mind can get when doing this flow before going to bed every night.

Getting started with **The Anti-Aging Flow (Right Side)**:
Step 1: Place your left fingers on your right cheekbone (left index finger where the cheek bone meets the edge of the right nostril, left middle and ring fingers flushed and on the cheekbone). Also, place your

right hand just below the right clav-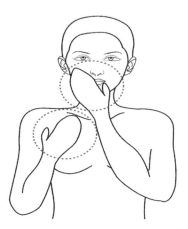
icle. I highly recommend that you
just clean out underneath the whole
clavicle area as this action will help
you to surrender to adapt to whatever environment you are dealing with
so that you won't have to fill your

head with all kinds of solutions. Breathe 3-4 breathing cycles.

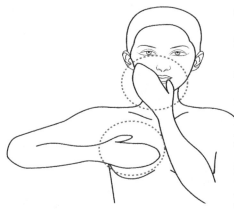

Step 2: Next, place the right
fingers a hand's-width from the
clavicle to the top of the breast
bone that is in alignment with
your right ear when your face
is facing completely forward.
Keep left fingers on the right

cheekbone. Breathe 3-4 breath cycles.

Step 3: Next, place right hand on the base of the front, left ribs (palming this area). Breathe 3-4 breath cycles.

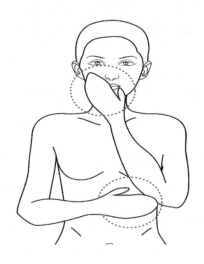

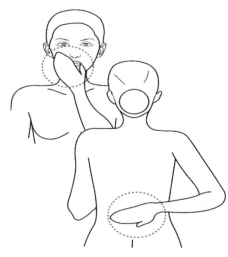

Step 4: Next, place the back of your right hand on the base of your left, back ribs (which means you will place your right hand on the left side near the small of your back on the left side). Left fingers remain on the right cheekbone. Breathe 3-4 deep breath cycles.

Step 5: Palm the base of the right, front ribs with your right hand while your left fingers stay in the anchoring position on the right cheekbone...and breathe 3-4 deep breath cycles.

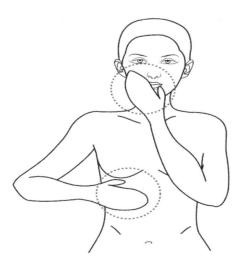

Step 6: Next, palm the inside (just above) the left knee with your right hand. Left fingers remain on the right cheekbone while you breathe deeply for 3-4 breath cycles.

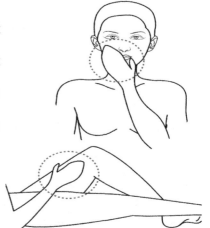

Step 7: Take your right hand and find the "eyes" of your left knee. Place your four right fingers together, excluding your thumb, about a hand's-width under your left knee bone. Your right baby finger should be touching just above the outer edge of your left shin bone. (Note:

left fingers remain in same position on right cheekbone.) Breathe deeply for 3-4 breath cycles.

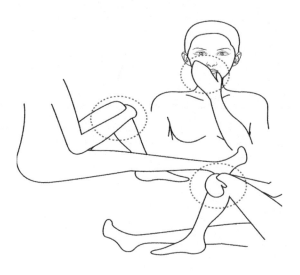

Step 8: Now, find the mid part of the left shin bone by measuring with your hands the halfway point between the left, inside ankle and the left knee. Place right hand here while the left fingers remain on the right

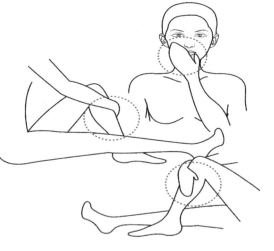

cheekbone. Breathe deeply for 3-4 breath cycles.

Step 9: Next, sandwich left, third toe with right thumb, index and middle fingers, while left fingers remain on the right cheekbone. Breathe deeply for 3-4 breath cycles, and afterwards release your hands and shake them out if you feel you need to.

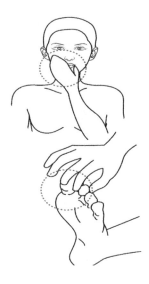

You can repeat the previous steps reversely for the Left Anti-Aging Flow (see Illustration 4 in the Appendix).

Chapter 10: Day 10
Eating Clean

I often hear people wanting to do internal cleanses to cleanse their internal organs. Yes, there are such things as a liver cleanse, a gallbladder cleanse, or even an intestinal cleanse. However, when you eat clean, you don't have to worry about doing this or that cleanse. What exactly does eating clean mean? It means that you eat food that is pesticide-free, organic (if possible), GMO free and full of wonderful nutrients. The following types of food DO NOT classify as "eating clean":

- *Fast food.* We don't know exactly what's in fast food!

- *Microwaved food.* The microwave should not be used for cooking or heating food. You can use the microwave to zap your dirty kitchen sponge of all the bacteria that is in it. The microwave is actually a modern device that is useless when it comes to your food. If it's not good for heating breast milk[1], what makes you think that it is good for you?

- *Processed food in a can or box.* If it's not natural, chances are it went through some heavy-duty process that requires chemicals and perhaps even some toxins. Not to mention,

---

1   Studies have shown that when you heat breast milk in the microwave, you are zapping away the nutrients.

the packaging could be very toxic. Preservatives used to keep that food edible is so not worth putting in your body.

- *TV dinners or food that is already cooked and frozen.* Many times, these foods are extremely high in sodium, and then people wonder why they are having a hard time shedding weight.

- *Junk food.* Whether that be a healthy version of chips or not! Make your own, like kale chips, or try eating dulse leaves which are packed with nutrients.

The main takeaway from this is that your food should be as natural as possible!

If you are an omnivore, then your animal products need to be organic, free-range and/or grass-fed (or wild for fish). Think about what animals naturally eat. Cows are not meant to eat grain, period. When they eat corn or things that they don't necessarily eat naturally, they can develop harmful bacteria in their gut, thus passing their gut issues to humans who eat them. As I'm sure you've heard before, you are what you eat!

Also, do your best to be GMO-free, and the easiest way to do that is to eat organic. Research has shown that genetically modified food has toxins that are passed into human blood matter and can interfere with our growth and development as human beings, especially in children. Not to mention the mere fact that, according to research published in the Public Library of Science, the mutations and fragments from GMO food can transfer from the digestive tract to the circulatory system within humans, thus linking it to cancer. Because GMOs are linked to exacerbating gluten sensitivities, you may choose to eat gluten-free if you're showing signs of any autoimmune symptom such as skin rashes, unexplained pain in the body, constant fatigue, breathing challenges, or chronic colds and flus.

Chapter 11: Day 11
Overcoming Sweet Cravings

S ugar comes in many forms, such as refined sugar, high fructose and corn syrup...basically, I'm naming all the bad forms of sugar. However, there are better alternatives to sugar such as stevia, honey, maple syrup or even dates. It's not that you should deny yourself of tasting sweetness, but choose wisely when satisfying your craving.

Before I share a hand pose to help you curb your sweet cravings, I want to share a story with you about a holistic practitioner friend of mine. She used to live down the street from a bakery. Whenever she would get a sweet craving, she would do this hand pose while walking to the bakery. She would often not have the sweet craving by the time she reached the bakery, thus turning her trip to the bakery into solely physical exercise and skipping the sweet treat.

Here's an illustration with the steps of what she used to do -

Left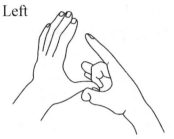

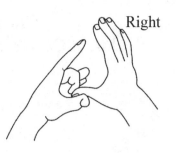 Right

Stack your right thumbnail on top of the pad of your left thumb, and then make a ring with your left middle finger so that the left middle fingernail touches the right thumb pad.

Hold for at least 9 breath cycles.

Stack your left thumbnail on top of the pad of your right thumb and then make a ring with your right middle finger so that the right middle fingernail touches the left thumb pad.

Again, hold for at least 9 breath cycles.

Do these daily and watch your sweet cravings diminish.

Chapter 12: Day 12
Rockin' Without the Toxins In Your Mind and Mouth

The next few days, I will be addressing toxicity in three different ways. Personally, I think this is the most important of all the "Rockin' Without the Toxins" days. This is about being mindful of your thoughts and what comes out of your mouth. Now, I'm not suggesting that you deny the physical truth, but I'm telling you that you have to look beyond the surface. I'm going to tell you about a recent epiphany I had about a family member because it changed my whole outlook of how I began to have more compassion for that family member. For years, I had issues with this family member; I was hurt by some of the things that I had heard were said about me behind my back. I basically cut this family member out of my life, temporarily, for at least 4 years. When I went to family gatherings, it was difficult because I could feel the energy of this family member feeling hurt as well. The truth is that I had abandoned her, and when she talked about me behind my back, I felt betrayed. So, I realized, my natural inclination is to want to abandon or reject before I am abandoned or rejected first. I was recently asked to join a group that this particular family member is already a part of and was seriously considering it. Even though I have come to terms with my relationship with her and the boundaries I've needed to draw around it, I became aware, as an empathic being, of my perspective of her. I felt like she was competitive and needed to be seen. Then, someone who isn't a part of our family said to me that they didn't see how this family member was competitive at all. Actually, she wants the best for all. I started to think how this could be true. How could I be wrong? I dove deeper and had a conversation with Spirit, and what I found was that this family member does what she does because she wants to be loved. It helped me to shed an even brighter light on this family member. It changed my toxic perception of her, and I saw the little girl who wants love just like ME.

Relationships can be challenging, and it is hard to keep out toxic thoughts and feelings with them because of our conditioning and experiences. As spirit beings, we come here to experience the world as a human being. It's in all the humanness that we begin to become discombobulated with life and how things should be. In my 53 years and metaphysical studies, Ralph Waldo Emerson is still my favorite metaphysician who I will always quote: "A man is what he thinks about all day long." Meaning, you are what you think. Your experience is what you think.

I believe, as humans, we strive to get as close as we can back to Source. The key is tapping into Source. As I mentioned in one of the earlier chapters, one of my yogi clients told me that the Vibrant Energy Flow System™ is plugging you into Source. I think of it as short-circuiting you back into Source. Sometimes it is difficult to believe all the affirmations that you say or want to manifest, but when you plug back into Source, you feel and know the Divine Truth. I am all about making life easy for you. So I have created the Detoxifying Flow - designed to help you diminish the toxic thoughts that breed fear and the physical manifestations of fear that show up in your body. So here, I present the Detoxifying Flow:

Directions for the **Right Detoxifying Flow:**

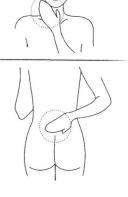

Step 1: Place your left hand on the right side of your neck. This is your anchor. Next, palm your tailbone with your right hand, and breathe about 9 breath cycles.

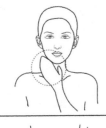

Step 2: Then, place your left fingers on your right sit bone (Note: if you bend your right knee, you will feel the sit bone if you are sitting or lying down). Breathe another 9 breath cycles.

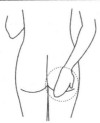

Step 3: Place your left fingers on the back of your right knee in the popliteal crease. This will help you with acute backaches and any feelings of not feeling supported or whatever fears that you may not even be conscious about. Breathe 9 breath cycles.

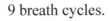

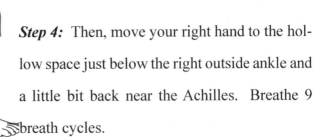

Step 4: Then, move your right hand to the hollow space just below the right outside ankle and a little bit back near the Achilles. Breathe 9 breath cycles.

Step 5: Next, your right hand goes on the out-side of the right cuboid bone; this is the lateral (outside) side of the foot just above the arch of the foot. Breath 9 breath cycles.

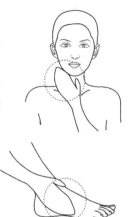

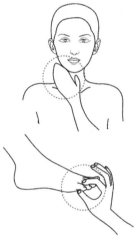

Step 6: Your final step is to allow your right fingers to sandwich your right baby toe and breathe.

Note how you feel, and you can repeat the steps reversely on the *left side* for the **Left Detoxifying Flow**:

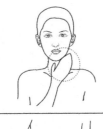

Step 1: Place your right hand on the left side of the neck. This is your anchor. Palm your tailbone with your left hand, and breathe about 9 breath cycles.

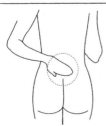

Step 2: Then, place your left fingers on your left sit bone (Note: if you bend your left knee, you will feel the sit bone if you are sitting or lying down). Breathe another 9 breath cycles.

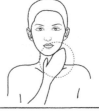

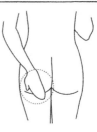

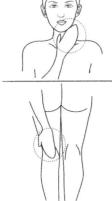

Step 3: Place your left fingers on the back of your left knee in the popliteal crease; this will help you with acute backaches and any feelings of not feeling supported or whatever fears that you may not even be conscious about. Breathe

9 breath cycles.

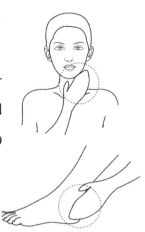

Step 4: Then, move your right hand to the hollow space just below the left outside ankle and a little bit back near the Achilles. Breathe 9 breath cycles.

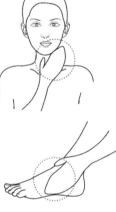

Step 5: Next, your left fingers touch the outside of the left cuboid bone; this is the lateral (outside) side of the foot just above the across the arch of the foot. Breathe 9 breath cycles.

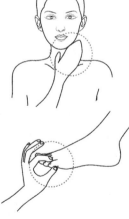

Step 6: Finally, allow your left fingers to sandwich the left baby toe, and breathe 9 breath cycles.

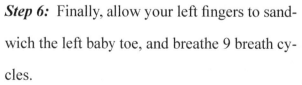

Chapter 13: Day 13
Rockin' Without the Toxins in Your Personal Temple

Your body is your God-given temple. You want to treat it with love and care so that your temple experiences longevity and vitality. It's time that you look at all the ingredients in your personal care products. For years, you may have been adding toxins to your own personal environment, your body. Your body is either confused by how to deal with those toxins, or it is fighting the battle to keep them at bay. It's time you look at your skincare and bodycare products. Do they have ingredients in them that you cannot pronounce, or do you even know all the ingredients in the product? Do they come from a trusted source? Really, you don't need all those products for your skin when some things from your kitchen suffice. For instance, avocado oil or even coconut oil can be used on the skin immediately after you bathe or shower. Lotion is nothing more than oil and water, so if you use the natural moisture on your skin with a good bottle of oil then you can achieve the same results as a bottle of lotion from your natural food store. Notice I didn't say a drug store; those lotions are already laced with all kinds of toxins. So here's the deal, it's very simple--parabens have been known to cause cancer, especially breast cancer--so avoid it in personal care products at all costs.

When I was a little girl, I watched my mom take care of her skin, so she served as a role model for me to begin my foundation of skincare. As I became a young lady myself, I evolved to using expensive skincare lines--which by the way, probably weren't the best for my skin--to now using natural, organic skincare that doesn't harm my skin at all. I found my current skincare line because of a breakout that I had after switching to my previous skincare line. I used to use Arbonne, but I didn't know all the ingredients in the line; besides, it was out of my budget, and the eye makeup remover burned my skin. No skincare products should burn your skin, especially your eyes. Today, I use coconut oil to remove my makeup. It is much gentler, doesn't burn, and does the first layer of cleansing without stripping my skin of any nutrients.

Everyone thinks that we want oil-free skincare. Many times, your skin breaks out because it lacks oil. I know because I was always using skincare as a teenager and young adult that would dry out my acne and make it worse. So if you think that your skin is going to break out because you put coconut oil on it, remember that coconut oil is antiviral.

Find an organic skincare product line. Just because it is organic doesn't mean that it is expensive. I highly recommend Luminance Skincare--you can find them online at http://www.luminanceskincare.com.

I also highly recommended avocado oil for the body. Here's why:

Avocado oil is a deeply penetrating oil that gets deep into the epidermis layers and moisturizes your skin like nobody's business. Aside from moisturizing your skin, it takes care of the fine lines and softens rough skin. It might be thick, but your skin absorbs it, and it doesn't leave an oily residue like coconut oil. The fatty acids in avocado oil are similar to the skin's own sebum, so it doesn't clog your pores.

Avocado oil is rich in healing vitamins B, C, D, E, K and especially, A (which increases cell-turnover), as well as potassium, lecithin, and chlorophyll. Avocado has compounds in it which are anti-inflammatory. Thus, avocado oil can help alleviate sun damage and age spots as well as skin conditions such as blemishes and eczema.

Moreover, avocado oil repairs the skin, thus giving it anti-aging benefits. It makes the skin more supple, elastic and resilient because it helps to increase the amount of collagen in the it.

Avocado oil offers low level UV protection as well, making it helpful for preventing sun damage; however, I do recommend that you use a non-toxic sunscreen in conjunction with it (and Luminance Skincare has one for you).

Finally, you can use it on your hair for an oil treatment or to oil your dry ends, bringing a nice sheen to your hair.

Chapter 14: Day 14
Rockin' Without the Toxins in Your Living and Work Environments

It's time to check all of your cleaning products, or rather, it is time to throw away and replace your cleaning products with non-toxic products. All those commercial products that might smell good and clean your clothes, your kitchen, your bathroom and your floors are leaking toxins into your system. When you breathe in all of those toxins, your lungs are ingesting them. Bleach and ammonia are a recipe for a toxic environment. Don't think the manufacturers of these type of cleaning products put warning labels on these products for fun. Those warnings are real. If you have lung problems, this could be the main reason why you have them. Your skin is the biggest lung on your body, so imagine what happens when you touch those products directly with your skin.

For many years since I turned into an adult at the age of 18, I battled asthma and many allergic reactions to the natural environment and my living and work environments. When I changed my cleaning products to a non-toxic environment, my allergies completely went away. For instance, the last house I rented had hardwood floors. I cleaned the floors with a water, Dr. Bronner's Castile Soap and olive oil solution instead of Murphy's Oil Soap. And the last time I painted my office, I used no-VOC paint to paint my walls. I remember my nephew who helped me telling me that it wasn't important, and after painting, he commented on how he didn't smell any chemicals and didn't get the woozy tired feeling from painting...because the paint was non-toxic.

You see, when we use non-toxic products in our environment, we diminish our health ailments to nothing by reducing the amount of toxins our bodies have to fight off and bringing our bodies back in balance. On that note, I'm going to give you a list of things you need to get started to put together a "clean home kit," so you can make your own products and disinfect things without harming yourself.

You might be thinking that that you paid good money for those toxic products...I bet you did. Understand that those toxic products are costing you your health in the long run? What if I told you that you will pay less for non-toxic products, and they will last longer? I still have a gallon of Dr. Bronner's Castile Soap that I purchased over a year ago.

Non-toxic cleaning kit:

- Dr. Bronner's Liquid Castile Soap
- Lemon essential oils
- Peppermint essential oils
- Baking soda - for scrubbing action
- Olive oil - for cleaning wood products
- Distilled water - for cleaning your fine wood furniture
- Hydrogen peroxide
- White distilled vinegar

You can find many DIY non-toxic cleaning recipes on the internet. Just do a search for DIY non-toxic cleaning products.

If you don't want to make your own cleaning products, here are my recommended non-toxic labels:

- Biokleen

- Seventh Generation
- Mrs. Meyers
- Ecos

Chapter 15: Day 15
Ease the Back

Your back supports you, and when you don't feel support-ed in your life, your back can actually give out on you. Sometimes it can be a dull pain that shows up slowly, or sometimes it can be a stabbing pain that shows up suddenly, like an earthquake just hit California.

Back pain takes a lot of energy out of you. It can also inhibit you from doing things that you may take for granted, like walking, exercising, or even driving. I remember in 2012, right when I was selling my home and dissolving my marriage, my back went out just two months before I was going to Machu Picchu, Peru, for a 10-day personal quest trip. I couldn't even WALK; I had to crawl around on my tile floors which was painful! I had to stop my weekly personal training exercise sessions so that I could heal my back. Sitting was even an issue for me and driving exasperated the pain. Of course, I went to my chiropractor--for heaven's sake, I shared an office with a bunch of them--plus I got this Vibrant Energy Flow System™ work done on me and did it myself as well. It's important to understand that my internal foundation was being shaken up even though I was the one who decided on ending the marriage. Plus, I think that it was God's way of telling me that I needed to enlist help to move, as in the past whenever we moved, I was the main one making sure that the house was packed up and waited for the movers while my 'was'-band enjoyed our alma mater's football game. This time Spirit said, 'No way you are going to take care of everyone once again!' I'm telling you this because I think that it is important for us to get to the root cause of our health ailments. What is going on emotionally and mentally plays a big part of the pain that we endure or the health ailment that we manifest.

Back pain can either be chronic (lasting for more than 90 days) or acute.

For acute back pain, hold behind your knees to help relieve the pain. Breathe about 36 breath cycles. This is an ancient healing method at work that helps relieve the pain quickly. You may need to do this more than once to allow all the pain to diminish. If the pain comes back, repeat as well. This inconspicuous hold is easy to do when you are watching a movie, lying down, sitting in a meeting, etc. No one is going to look at you and ask why you're holding behind your knees.

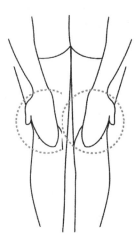

For chronic pain (lasting more than 90 days, even if it comes and goes), you want to hold the area just below the lateral ankle and slightly back towards the Achilles in the hollow space there, and breathe for 36 breath cycles.

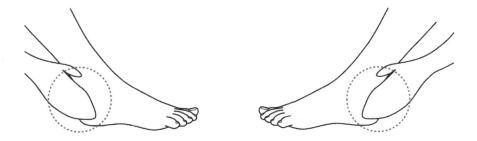

I encourage you to share how this works for you because back pain can be one of the most stubborn aches to deal with.

Here's another hint: When dealing with back pain, consider what emotion may be activating the pain. It is usually FEAR. What are you fearful about? Where are you not showing up courageously in your life? You might want to take a journal and write down your thoughts about this.

Also, to ensure that back pain doesn't overtake you, the De-toxifying Flow from Chapter 12 can also help alleviate immediate back pain or can be used as a preventative measure to avoid future back pain.

Chapter 16: Day 16
Happiness = Vibrancy

If you are a person who can always make the best out of any situation, then you are probably considered a Pollyanna. It's a good thing; it means that you don't let the world get you down. Now, this doesn't mean that you let people walk all over you or that you have no boundaries. Rather, it means that you find the good in every situation, even if it just means that you learned a lesson from it.

If you are a person like the archetype Eeyore (the sad donkey from Winnie the Pooh), who is always expecting the worst to happen, then the worst is what shows up in your life.

We can't let the conditions we picked up from our family and the world's consciousness lead. When they lead, you can fall ill. I see it all the time--a person eats well, exercises and takes care of themselves well, but then they fall ill to a scary label like cancer. Then we question, why is it that the person who smokes and drinks lives longer?

Sometimes I have to ask if the rigidity of eating clean is too much for a person. Some people feel that in order to stay healthy you have to suffer by eating healthy food that tastes bad and doesn't give you joy. But that isn't true in this modern day! You can enjoy vegan desserts that are actually packed with wonderful nutrients and still taste good. It's also important to consider how the food was prepared. Was it prepared with joy, or was it prepared with anger? Everything, including food preparation, is energy. It can leave you feeling happy and joyful or with a stomachache that hits you suddenly and leaves you with food poisoning.

Exercise can also be done with joy. Are you exercising because you think you have to, or is exercise something you enjoy doing in your life? For instance, I hike almost 3 times a week, sometimes daily. I do it to commune with nature; it is a Spiritual ritual for me, but I also gain benefits from the hiking. Another way that I exercise with joy is through dance. My inner child loves to dance! I grew up in a dancing family. Any opportunity we had at a family gathering, we would put on the music and start grooving. In my heart, those were good times of joy and laughter for me. So, I take dance classes at least twice a week to feed my inner child who loves to dance. Of course, I also benefit from the movement and aerobic exercise dancing provides for my 50-something body.

What you project onto the world is your experience and it reflects in your way of being and how you age. What are you projecting onto the world in this moment? Is it what you want reflected back to you?

The Vibrant Energy Flow System™ is great for changing your outlook on life. I had a client who once shared with me how her relationship with her father, who she couldn't stand for many years, had recently changed. She didn't make any direct effort to change her relationship with him and realized that The Vibrant Energy Flow System™ had rewired her attitude towards him.

Many modalities talk about how you rewire the neurotransmitters. The same thing happens with the Vibrant Energy Flow System™.

Here's a challenge to help you boost happiness and vibrancy - Do one of the Vibrant Energy Flows daily and watch how your vibrancy shifts with how you react to things in your life.

Chapter 17: Day 17
Look Under the Hood
of Your Attitude

Many of the health challenges that we encounter come from our emotions and attitude towards life. You might disagree with me because science always points it to genetics. What if I told you that attitudes are passed down through generations and that many times you inherit your attitude from the generations before you? As you can see, I am digging deeper now. I like to dig into what's really going on with you. I don't mean to pry, but if we can get to the heart of what might be causing any distress in your body, then together we can probably improve your life expectancy and quality.

When I first started studying the healing arts, I was given a hand chart of attitudes which I have now made into my own and expanded to include the body systems and energies affected. I will now pass the chart onto you via my website

http://www.selfcarequeendom.com.

Many who know meridians from Chinese Medicine might be

confused by the chart, but this chart goes beyond the meridians and looks at the source of the attitudes. So this chart will help you on a cosmic level, whereas the meridians work on the physical level (even though you can't touch them). It's a good place to start and can help you have a state change in your emotions and behavior, especially when you lose your cool or you find yourself fretting over one of the attitudes indicated on the chart.

When I first started practicing the healing arts, I had a girl-friend who had been a co-worker from the hi-tech industry. She found it difficult getting pregnant and had encountered a series of miscar-riages. One day while working on her, she informed me that she had trouble falling asleep. I asked her what seemed to be the problem. She told me that she would always think about all the things she had to do the next day for her job. Immediately, I intuited that this had to do with the attitude of worry. I gave her a homework assignment to hold her thumbs when going to bed at night. At her next session, she reported to me that she did her homework as instructed and found herself still holding her thumbs when she awakened the next morning. She was amazed that not only did it work, but she got great sleep.

If you haven't done this already, go to my Self-Care Queendom website (http://www.selfcarequeendom.com) and download the special report - "The Five Attitudes that Keep You from Having Vibrant Health & Energy." This special report includes the hand chart and an audio guide instructing you how to use it. Even better, go to my YouTube channel to see a video of how to use this chart at https://youtu.be/cmQ53R3qRGE.

Chapter 18: Day 18
Healthy Breasts

How could something so nurturing for our babies turn into something that could possibly take your life away? There are a lot of things linked to breast cancer, including radiation exposure. The best risk-free assessment tool for your breasts is thermography. Notice I didn't say a mammogram. Thermography is a safe, proven method to detect cancer via hotspots in your body, whereas mammograms expose you to the very thing that can cause cancer, radiation. Our environment is already buzzing with enough exposure to radiation, so why put radiation directly onto your body?

Personally, I like to focus on having healthy breasts. So, I continue to do flows from the Vibrant Energy Flow System™ to help clear any blocks that may appear as tumors or cysts in the body. Here's a flow you can do that will help you clear any attitude that might cause breast cancer, such as resentment, unworthiness, or not feeling nurtured. Check out my healthy breast flow:

Place your right hand on the upper area of your left arm. Now,

take your left hand and place it just above the
inside of your right knee, and breathe for 9
breath cycles.

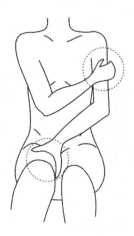

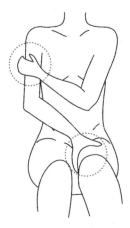

Now, do the opposite side. Place left hand on the
upper area of your right arm and place your right
hand just above the inside of your left knee, and
breathe 9 breath cycles.

As we age, women become more concerned about our breasts
sagging. I highly recommend the following breast oil by Rupam's
Herbals; not only does it help to firm up your breasts, but it also helps
with any fibrocystic tissues (http://www.rupamherbals.com/#!prod-
uct/prd2/4415961031/lady-nada's-breast-oil-1.5-oz).

Chapter 19: Day 19
Calm your Nerves

Feeling overwhelmed, anxious, and being a perfectionist share a common thread with each other. Unfortunately, we live in a society of "keeping up with the Joneses." I admit to falling into this trap myself, especially when I was a young parent trying to keep up with the rest of the parents. I think it's something many of us naturally find ourselves doing as young parents. By fifty, when my nest was empty, I stopped caring about what people thought of me anymore. However, I see that anxiety and overwhelm run rampant in our society. What exactly does this look like? Perhaps, you can't finish a project because it just isn't good enough. I think that, as a society that judges based on grades, test scores and what college you get into, we promote this bullshit of perfection. I ask, what are we modeling for our young ones? Is this what happiness is really all about?

So here's what you can do to calm your nerves and to stop all the feelings of anxiety and overwhelm--there's a point on your wrist that can change the state of your anxiety in less than 60 seconds. Just touch the palm side of your left wrist on top of the baby finger side of your right fingers, and breathe 36 breath cycles. Relax your shoulders and feel your body begin to relax and feel your heartbeat slow down.

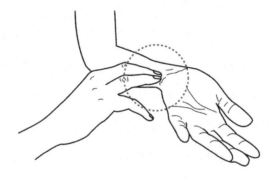

It's that easy to calm your nerves. I'd love to hear how this quick energy release flow has helped you. Please share in the Vibrant Energy Flow System Facebook Group (https://www.facebook.com/groups/30day2avibranthealthieryoungeryou/).

Chapter 20: Day 20
Having More Stamina

These days, I hear all the time about the "tiredness" epidemic. So many of us live as human "doings" instead of human "beings" that we forget to rest, and then we end up tapping out our energy reserves. So, I'm going to teach you how to have more stamina.

First of all, the Anti-Aging Flow (Illustration 4 in the Appendix) has a point in the flow pattern that helps you have more stamina. So, if you do this flow on yourself daily (on at least one side), you will help yourself have more stamina. But here's another quick one for you that I used while I was in Peru, hiking at high altitudes that I wasn't used to. It's a simple hand pose that you can do. First, make a ring with your thumbs and ring fingers on each side so that your thumb pads touch the nails of your ring fingers like the illustration:

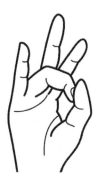 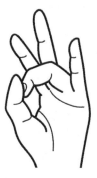

Be sure to breathe at least 9 breath cycles as you hold each finger, and notice how much more relaxed you feel. Also, notice how the tension in your body diminishes.

Chapter 21: Day 21
Unclogging the Sinuses

Often, I hear from clients and from owners of my DVD product, *30 Days to a Vibrant, Healthier, Younger You,* that people are having problems with sinus congestion. This may look like their nose is running profusely, or they feel like they can't breathe through their nostrils. Many experience headaches in the sinus cavity, which may feel like a lot of pressure on top of the nose, between your eyebrows. Many experience sinus pressure on either or both sides of the nostrils near the cheek bones.

First of all, I'm going to tell you what I tell my clients: If you have chronic nasal congestion, then chances are that you have candida. This is a sign that you need to adjust your lifestyle habits to eliminate gluten, dairy, and any sugars from your diet. Candida requires very strict practices to heal, but you will love the results once you get over the die-off of candida albicans.

When I first discovered this work, I had horrible springtime allergies. Even though I had the Vibrant Energy Flow System™, I still had a touch of asthma flare up every now and then, and my sinuses still ran profusely, intermittently, even though they were improved in the spring. The Vibrant Energy Flow System™ alone was not enough to expel such an extreme health challenge that I had for decades. It was when I truly stopped eating gluten, dairy, and sugar, that my allergies cleared up. I didn't experience any more sinus congestion.

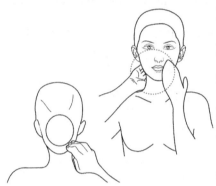

However, the quick tip that I share with people to immediately release sinus congestion is to put your right hand on the base of your right skull (occipital ridge), and put your left fingers on the left cheekbone, as close as you can get to the edge of the left nostril.

Because this is a bilateral concept, you want to repeat this on the opposite side--left hand on the base of the left skull (occipital ridge) and right hand on the right cheek bone.

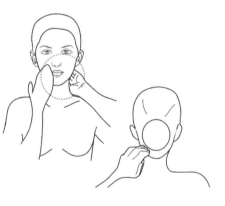

If you really want to help relieve your allergies, cross your arms and place your finger pads right underneath your collar bone (clavicle). Actually, I suggest that you clear it out from the edge of where the clavicle meets the shoulder-arm joint (anatomically known as the glenohumeral joint) to the either side of the sternum (the neck-tie-looking bone that connects your left and right breast bone ribs). Ahhh....and breath nine to thirty-six breath cycles.

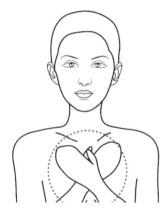

Again, I would love it if you shared your results within the Vibrant Energy Flow System Facebook Group (https://www.facebook.com/groups/30day2avibranthealthieryoungeryou/).

Chapter 22: Day 22
Optimize Your Exercise

I am now going to help you to be wise about your exercise. You see, I'm all about you enjoying your exercise. It's not about hitting the grind just to have a hot body, but let's get your exercise to work for you...or even get your non-exercise to work for you. This is all about regenerating your cells. Here's how you do it:

After exercising, the best way to get your exercise to work for you is to simply sit on your hands (making sure your fingers are touching your sit bones) and just breathe about 36 breath cycles. This helps your cells to regenerate, thus optimizing your exercise.

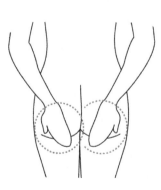

Chapter 23: Day 23
ReSet Your Inner Clock

This is wonderful if you've been traveling to a different time zone and you need to acclimate yourself instead of experiencing jet lag. Or, this can even work when we spring our clocks ahead for daylight savings time in the spring or turn them back in the fall.

So, what you want to do is place your left hand on your right shoulder and your right hand on your right sit bone. Then, breathe about 36 breath cycles.

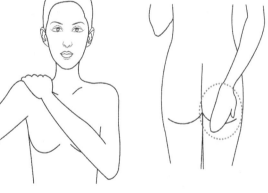

Reverse sides by placing your right hand on your left shoulder and your left fingers on your left sit bone, and breathe 36 breaths again.

If you find your-self waking up in the middle of the night be-cause your internal clock hasn't synced up with the new time zone, then this is also a great thing to do.

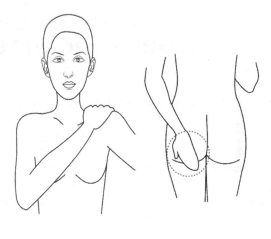

I had a client who traveled to Egypt (from the San Francisco Bay Area) for 10 days of vacation. When she returned home, she was super jetlagged. She would be wide awake at night when she needed to be sleeping and ready to sleep during the daytime. Well, that didn't work too well for her because she was an IT consultant for a company in the financial district and she needed to be "on" for her work. When she came to me, I simply worked on the self-help quick release pattern that I just gave you. The next day she left me a voicemail telling me how she had gotten the best night of sleep, and she didn't wake up at 3 AM like she had done before. I had re-set her body clock, and you can do this too for yourself when you are experiencing jet lag, daylight savings time adjustment, standard time adjustment in the fall, or just simply insomnia. Sometimes our body needs to be reminded about the internal body clock it has.

When daylight savings time comes around, the owners of the *30 Days to a Vibrant, Healthier, Younger You* Video Product who do these flows regularly do not have issues adjusting to the time change.

Chapter 24: Day 24
Letting Go of the Pain in the Neck

L iving day to day, most of us feel the need to want to control everything in our lives. We even want to control the behavior of other people, especially of our children. Our bodies wreak havoc of wanting to be in control of everything in our lives. Most often it shows up in our necks. The neck is either pained (because we feel that someone is being a pain in the neck…because they aren't doing what we think or want them to do) or we awaken to not being able to turn our neck. Most often this type of case is blamed on the way that we slept or our pillow caused it. When our necks can't move freely, we are being rigid about a situation or about everything in our lives. Often I'll ask a person, what are they angry about or who is a pain in the neck? Everyone could use some neck releasing. The pain and stiffness that shows up in the neck is usually how people show up with their control freak selves. Yes, even I'm guilty of it. So now I'm going to give you a quick release flow to help you relax and relinquish control.

So, right now, just take the time to put your right hand on the right side of your neck and your left hand on your right upper arm, and breathe 36 breaths. Note what you feel. For those who feel like they have to do - do to control life, this is a great opportunity for you to release the need to sit in generating energy like the "Energizer Bunny" that keeps going and going.

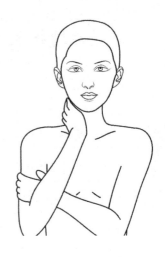

One day while I was doing this quick release on myself, I fell asleep while I got really warm; it was the same warmness I feel when I work on clients while they are doing some deep energetic releasing.

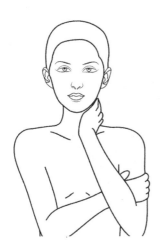

If you find yourself feeling like you have to manipulate others to get what you want, place your left hand on the left side of your neck and hold the upper part of your left arm with your right hand, and breathe 36 breaths.

After doing this quick release, I would love to hear how it felt for you physically, mentally and emotionally. You will want to report your findings in the Vibrant Energy Flow System Facebook Group (https://www.facebook.com/groups/30day2avibranthealthieryoungeryou/). When you share what happens to you, you give us more inspiration, more proof, more data...you touch another soul in some way shape or form.

Chapter 25: Day 25
The Skinny on Essential Fatty Acids

L et's get straight on essential fatty acids because this is a big one to increase your longevity. Many already know that you need to have Omega-3, 6 and 9, but they are unaware of the ratios. Not knowing the proper ratios can actually do more harm than good.

Omega-3 and Omega-6 are considered essential fatty acids that we can only get from food. Omega-9 can be manufactured in your body from our food, but doesn't necessarily have to be consumed exclusively. A good ratio for Omega-6 to Omega-3 is between 1:1 and 4:1. Unfortunately, many of us over consume Omega-6 thus resulting in an Omega-6 to Omega-3 ratio of 10:1 - 25:1, making you Omega-3 deficient. Such an imbalance of EFAs has been linked to many health challenges including depression, heart attacks, cancer, insulin resistance, asthma, lupus, schizophrenia, postpartum depression, accelerated aging, stroke, obesity, diabetes, arthritis, ADHD, and Alzheimer's Disease, among others.

Here's the key - One tablespoon of flaxseed OIL (not seeds) is sufficient enough to provide you with the right balance of Omega-6 to Omega-3 per day. Flaxseed oil cannot be heated, but it can be used in a salad dressing or put on warm food (not hot). The body will synthesize the right amount of Omega-9 from such a source. Omega-6 is found in many of our daily foods including flaxseed oil, flaxseeds, flaxseed meal, hempseed oil, hemp seeds, grape seed oil, pumpkin seeds, pine nuts, pistachio nuts, sunflower seeds (raw), olive oil, olives, borage oil, evening primrose oil, black currant seed oil, chestnut oil, and chicken. You want to avoid refined and hydrogenated versions of these foods at all costs. These may show up in corn, safflower, sunflower, soybean, and cottonseed oils.

My suggestions for maximum oil consumption in a day are as follows:

- If you feel that you could release some weight – none or very little; you may only take Omega-3 oils and Gamma Linolenic Acid (GLA), which is classified as an Omega-6 fatty acid.
- If you feel like you could use some extra weight, then consume up to one tablespoon of Omega-3 oil.

- If you feel that you don't have any particular weight im-balances, then one teaspoon is plenty to consume of Ome-ga-3 oils.

Most foods can be cooked without oils and that's the way that I generally cook all of my foods.

Unrefined monounsaturated oils generally are healthy. They are recommended for those who have too much stored fat and choles-terol – most who eat large amounts of animal protein. I recommend olive oil from the West and sesame oil from the East.

Olive oil is recommended as a great monounsaturated fat for salad dressings and for giving foods flavor after cooking them. It is not recommended for cooking because when heated, it is susceptible to creating free radical cells (oxidative damage). Take a look at the top three grades: Extra virgin olive oil is recommended because it has a maximum acidity of 1%. Fine virgin olive oil is next at 1.5% and then current virgin at 3%. However, make sure the oils are always organic and unrefined.

Sesame oil is both monounsaturated and polyunsaturated, fif-ty-fifty. Normally we would expect the polyunsaturated portion to quickly become rancid, but it is a very stable oil because as an antioxidant – sesamol is naturally present in it.

When cooking at high temperatures – clarified butter and coconut oil are recommended.

Clarified butter, which is sometimes called ghee, is butter with milk solids removed, thus containing butyric acid, a fatty acid that has antiviral and anticancer properties; it has also been found to be helpful when preventing and treating Alzheimer's disease. Might I add that clarified butter enhances an essence that governs the tissues and balances the hormones. Ghee is a staple among Ayurvedic cooking; it is very useful for those who have depleted their kidney jing (essence) by excessive sexual activity and can help restore the kidney jing (essence). It is great for increasing digestive fire, which improves assimilation thus enhancing the nutritional value received from foods.

Coconut oil is a powerful virus destroyer and antibiotic just like ghee/clarified butter, but is a vegan/vegetarian option. It is a saturated fat that contains lauric acid. Lauric acid has unique healing properties; your body converts lauric acid into monolaurin, which has anti-viral, anti-bacterial and anti-protozoa properties. According to natural health expert Dr. Joseph Mercola, coconut oil contains the most lauric acid of any substance on Earth.

Some of the benefits of coconut oil are:

- Promotes heart health - important during perimeno-pause and menopause
- Promotes weight loss – very important when we are going through perimenopause
- Supports a healthy metabolism
- Provides you with an immediate energy source
- Keeps your skin radiantly healthy and youthful
- Supports the proper function of thyroid gland
- Helps with the immune system

Coconut oil is a 2/3 medium chain fatty acid (MCFA) known as medium-chained triglycerides or MCTs. The benefits of MCFAs are:

- They permeate your cell membranes easily, unlike the long

chain fatty acids (LCFAs) that most vegetable and seed oils are comprised of.

- They are easily digested, thus putting less strain on your digestive system.
- They are sent directly to your liver, where they are immediately converted into energy rather than being stored as FAT.
- They stimulate your body's metabolism.

Coconut oil fights diabetes by not producing an insulin spike in your body….and yes it can help prevent diabetes.

Here are some ways for you to get the proper balance of the EFAs:

- Take a teaspoon of High Lignan Flaxseed Oil. (The maximum is 1 tablespoon, depending on your weight. The more overweight you are, the less oil you need to consume.)
- Eat an avocado every day. I myself replace mayonnaise on a sandwich or burger with avocado. Avocados satisfy the Omega-3 requirement. This is you making healthier choices in your life instead of going for the norm. Give yourself nutrients naturally with your food.

- Eat dark leafy vegetables daily, such as kale, collards, spinach, or mustard greens.
- Snack on nuts, such as walnuts, pumpkin seeds, or Brazil nuts.
- If you are an omnivore who consumes fish, then make sure you eat some wild Omega-3 rich fish such as salmon, mackerel, sardines and anchovies, albacore tuna or black cod (butterfish).

Chapter 26: Day 26
Aging Gracefully

Aging is a natural process that our body does as we experience our solar return each year. How we age is up to how we use our body's energies. In Chinese Medicine, it is believed that we are given a finite amount of energy to live out this life in this particular body that we have been given. How we use that energy depends on the longevity of someone's life. If we run around stressed out all the time, then we will age quickly. Our daily life habits have an influence on how we age. If you smoke or drink alcohol excessively, then you will show signs of aging earlier in life. Our grey hairs are just one way that we all show age. In Chinese Medicine, the following habits can age you quickly:

- For men, excessive ejaculation; hence, this is why many men experience erectile dysfunction as they age

- For women, too many pregnancies or little time to recover between pregnancies; this is why we often see exhausted, super busy moms

- High stress that's taxing on the adrenals, which later shows up during menopause as hot flashes and insomnia, but can also affect your ability to conceive a child

- Thrilling activities like riding a rollercoaster

If you learn to go with the flow, life will be easier on you, and you won't see as many signs of aging.

It's important to recognize signs of premature aging and nip them in the bud before they take over:

- Back pain
- Knee pain
- Frequent urination
- Hair greying
- Energy reserves feeling tapped out

Doing the Vibrant Energy Flows religiously could help you prevent premature aging. For sure, it will shift your perception of life and change your relationship to it. Over time, you might find yourself reacting to people and situations differently, thus helping you to go with the flow of life.

Today, make a decision to commit yourself to doing all five of the flow patterns given to you. You don't have to do all of them every day, but choose at least one or two flows to do each day. I have clients who do one flow at night like the Anti-Aging Flow to release the mental activity for the day, then they do the Energizing Flow first thing in the morning to make sure they have focused energy. Pick a flow to do each day, or do all five flows if you have time in the morning. Each flow can take up to twenty minutes, but in general all five flows only take an hour of your time. When you have a little bit more time on a weekend, you might want to do all five flows in one sitting. Commit to it and watch it change your life.

Chapter 27: Day 27
Loving Yourself Totally

L oving yourself unconditionally is one of the best gifts you can give yourself. Wrap your arms around yourself, look in the mirror and tell yourself how much you love you. Here's the truth, when we love ourselves by showing it, we can be there to support our people, tribe, friends, and most of all, our family.

When you commit to doing the Vibrant Energy Flow System™ it is a form of love that you give yourself so you can be there for your peeps. Knowing that, which Vibrant Energy Flow will you commit to today? It's your choice! Centering, Attitude Adjustment, Energizing, Anti-Aging or Detoxifying Flow. Remember, for those four flows that are bilateral, you only have to do one side. Which side will you choose? Choose based on your needs - emotional vs. lifestyle. If you are feeling emotional, then the left side is probably a great place for you to start. If you are trying to kick or change a habit, then the right side is a good place to go. Otherwise, just listen to your body and go to the side that calls you. For all of the flows, please see the Appendix.

Don't Touch My Body

I added this chapter because I had a client and friend, Ruby, who got to a point where she said that she had to take a break from doing the Vibrant Energy Flows on her body for about six months or so. You probably have seen her before-and-after pictures on some of my promotional material. Even I have felt that I've sometimes needed to take a break. So the question arises, what do you do when you feel like your body just doesn't want to be touched by yourself? It's a good time to find a practitioner to help you, or what I do is the mudras (hand poses).

Sometimes your body doesn't feel like being touched, or sometimes your hands don't feel like touching your body. You can continue to receive the Vibrant Energy Flow System™, but with hand poses known as mudras. Borrowed from the Eastern philosophies of Hinduism and Buddhism, mudras are body poses that have an influence on the energies of the body or mood, using solely the hands and fingers. Most people are familiar with these hand poses when meditating. To get you started, here are eight hand poses you can do daily to bring your body's energies back into balance.

CENTERING MUDRAS
Part I

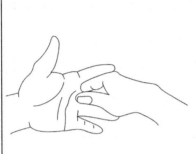	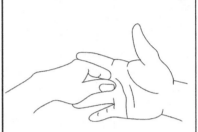
Left side: Hold the palm side of your left middle finger lightly with your right thumb. Place rest of right fingers on the back of left middle finger.	*Right side:* Hold the palm side of your right middle finger lightly with your left thumb. Place rest of right fingers on the back of left middle finger.

This first hand pose can help you to exhale and let go. It is also a finger to hold when you find yourself angered by a situation. It helps to diminish anger and balance hormones. It also helps improve vision, both physically and spiritually (via the third eye between the eyebrows).

Part II

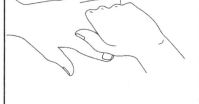

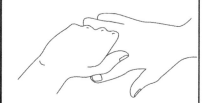

Left side: Hold back of left middle finger lightly with right thumb. Place rest of right fingers on palm side of left middle finger.

Right side: Hold back of right middle finger lightly with left thumb. Place rest of left fingers on palm side of right middle finger.

The second hand pose can help you breathe deeper by allowing more oxygen/air to get into your air passage way. It also helps you to RECEIVE. Again, because it is the middle finger that you are holding, anger will continue to diminish, allowing you to feel a much more vulnerable feeling behind your anger. Note: the first two hand poses are equivalent to the CENTERING FLOW.

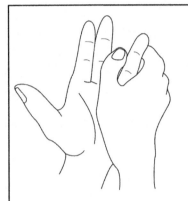

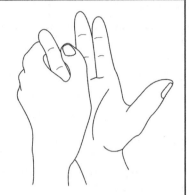

Left side: Hold palm side of left little and ring fingers with right thumb. Place rest of right fingers on the back of left little and ring fingers.

Right side: Hold palm side of right little and ring fingers with left thumb. Place rest of left fingers on the back of right little and ring fingers.

This hand pose helps to calm the body down by releasing tension along the full spectrum of emotions ranging from sadness, grief and depression to nervous, yet joyful laughter.

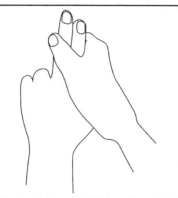

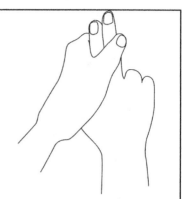

Left side: Hold back of left thumb, index and middle fingers with right thumb. Place rest of right fingers on palm side of the left thumb, index and middle fingers.

Right side: Hold back of right thumb, index and middle fingers with left thumb. Place rest of left fingers on palm side of the right thumb, index and middle fingers.

Call it what you will, but this is a powerhouse finger pose, helping you to release your daily stresses of worries, fears, and anger. Ever find yourself irritable? Do this finger pose and breath for 18 breaths on each side. This is the anti-aging finger pose; after all, it melts away those three critical stresses that age us....right?

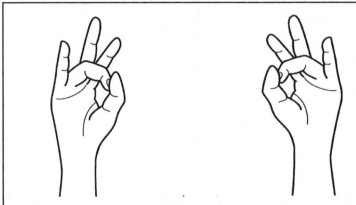

Both sides: Touch the ring fingernail with the same side thumb pad (palm side). Do both sides simultaneously.

This mudra is known for its ability to improve stamina because it helps you to breathe easier when exercising. It can also be used at high altitudes while flying or driving and is great to use on airplane trips and trips to the mountains.

ENERGIZING MUDRA

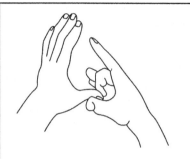 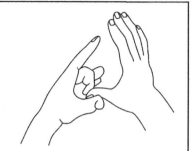

Left side: Stack the left thumbnail on top of the right thumb pad and then stack right middle fingernail on top of the left thumb pad by making a circle with it.	*Right side:* Stack the right thumbnail on top of the left thumb pad and the left middle fingernail on top of the right thumb pad by making a circle with it.

The energizing mudra is great to help you bust through sugar cravings. It makes sense, right? You crave sweet stuff like candy, pastries and simple carbohydrates when you need a quick "pick me up." This mudra helps us get energy from our food more efficiently and helps us take in nutritious food.

HARMONY MUDRA

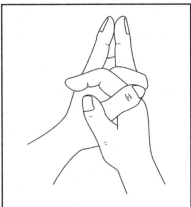

Fold your hands and touch the palms of the left and right middle fingers.

The harmony mudra brings balance to our total being. If you notice, it's like we are praying, but with the two middle fingers touching. This mudra help us to release daily tension from head to toe, throughout our entire physiology, including our digestive, respiratory, eliminatory, and endocrine systems. It aids in releasing all of the day's energies that you may have absorbed or experienced. One of my senior clients uses this mudra to put herself to sleep at night.

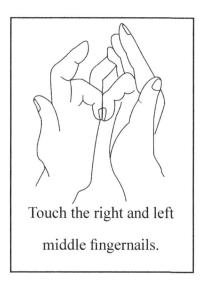

Touch the right and left
middle fingernails.

The relieve-the-stress mudra is indicative of its name. It is strongly associated with the centering flow and can be another mudra used to substitute for doing the entire centering flow. This mudra relieves back stress and helps one breathe easier.

Chapter 29: Day 29
A State Change

When I was in college, I studied and earned a degree in electrical engineering. One of the classes that I took was a computer science class that showed us how Boolean logic worked and how we could change states quickly. The same is true as we apply the Vibrant Energy Flow System™ to our human bodies. Our human bodies are like computers. They have all kind of systems--the bones, the muscles, the blood, the glandular system, the endocrine system, the organs, and so on. Our bodies become disharmonized from reactions to situations or experiences of the past (whether that be this lifetime or a past life, if you believe in that). Our DNA holds patterns from our ancestors, and we can choose to go that route or not; sometimes, unconsciously, it happens and we don't understand or know that we are following their footsteps. Is it karma? Especially if you are named after a grandparent or aunt, it makes you wonder how much that affects how you appear in this world.

Everything is Energy. The Vibrant Energy Flow System™ embodies you as the jumper cable, recharging and restoring your body's energy. It provides a state change for you (an opportunity for you to change the disharmonized state of being to one that is Divine in nature) and reminds you who you really are in the eyes of the Universe. So when you are applying this healing art, it is so much more than just acupressure or shifting your health; it has a spiritual aspect to it as well. It is exactly that spiritual aspect that makes your heart beat its natural rhythm instead of the fast and heavy beat that happens when you feel overwhelmed, panicked or anxious. It helps your lungs grasp oxygen efficiently instead of feeling like air will not get into your air passageway, thus allowing you to breathe deeper and with ease. It can help your pancreas to make insulin naturally after it has been overused because your body has been fed too much food high in sugar content. The Vibrant Energy Flow System™ reminds you who you are, even if you don't feel the effects yet because you might have such a severe disharmony of the body. There are no side effects. You can't mess up. You can't overdose. Sometimes you have to wait for your body to take it in, and you have to keep reprogramming your body until your body remembers the truth of who it is, because it is natural for it to slip back to the disharmonized state that it has been in for a long time. That's why doing these five flow patterns daily or substituting with the mudras will help you have the state change that you would like to experience in body, mind and Spirit. Ask yourself, what state change do you want to experience? Then choose at least one flow pattern if you can't do all of them daily. The flow patterns are named purposely by how they will serve you best.

The Centering Flow (see Appendix, Illustration 1)

- Centers you
- Brings your hormones back into balance
- Supports the immune system
- Can improve your sleep
- Can calm you quickly

The Attitude Adjustment Flow (see Appendix, Illustration 2)

- Can help you shift your emotions and/or attitude
- Can help you get rid of your emotional or even unconscious DNA baggage
- Can help you shift a perspective
- Helps with depression
- Helps relieve tension in shoulders

The Energizing Flow (see Appendix, Illustration 3)

- Energizes you

- Helps you focus

- Helps to balance your blood sugar levels

- Converts your food efficiently into energy

- Can help with bloating

The Anti-Aging Flow (See Appendix, Illustration 4)

- Helps smooth out the wrinkles in your face from all the reactions to life

- Increases your stamina

- Has been known to reverse gray hairs

- Helps release mental stress

- Calms a monkey mind

- Can relieve a frontal headache

- Helps to balance appetite

The Detoxifying Flow (See Appendix, Illustration 5)

- Helps you detox your body, mentally and physically

- Helps relieve a backache

- Reduces frequent urination

- Relieves tension in shoulders

- Relieves a back-of-the-head headache

Chapter 30: Day 30
Take the Bait &
Just Meditate

L et's be clear -- this practice is your meditation. Oftentimes, people have a hard time quieting their mind to meditate. This system helps you to quiet your mind with ease. If you want to take the next step and not have to think about what you are doing and be guided, you might want to just take the plunge and purchase the virtual product, which includes instructional videos, guided audios (which are different from the videos), and 30 emails that help you embody this work. It's truly life changing once you embrace it. I've had people resist and keep their same disharmonies, and I've had people embrace it and see what a difference it has made in their lives.

I keep hearing what my yogi friend said to me years ago, when she first experienced this work: "It's plugging you into Source." Why not get yourself plugged into Source? So just take the bait and meditate...it can't hurt you; it can only help you! You can purchase the virtual product, *30 Days to a Vibrant, Healthier, Younger You* at http:// www.selfcarequeendom.com/30days.

Stay tuned for even more flows, and get the 30 Days to a Vibrant Healthier Younger You plus more with the *Vibrant Energy Flow System™ 2.0 Home Study Program.* Register here for the program - *Vibrant Energy Flow System™ 2.0 Home Study Program* (http://selfcarequeendom.com/vefs2-0-offer/).

APPENDIX

ILLUSTRATION 1
CENTERING FLOW

Benefits

- *Aids balancing hormones*

- *Centers you*

- *Grounds you*

- *Builds immune system*

- *Helps with restful sleep*

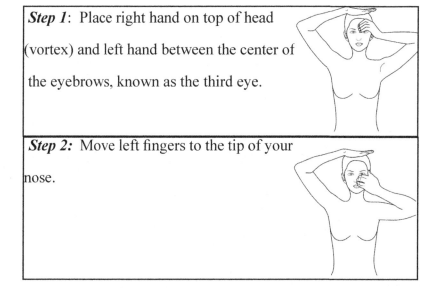

Step 1: Place right hand on top of head (vortex) and left hand between the center of the eyebrows, known as the third eye.
Step 2: Move left fingers to the tip of your nose.

Step 3: Place left index finger on the philtrum (indentation between the upper lip and the nose), and the left middle and ring fingers touch the indentation between the lower lip and the chin.

Step 4: Place the left fingers in between the indentation right above where the sternum and left and right clavicle meet (near the throat).

Step 5: Place the left fingers in the middle of the breasts, right on the sternum.

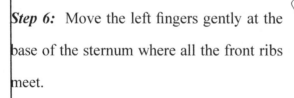
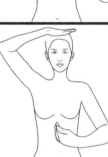

Step 6: Move the left fingers gently at the base of the sternum where all the front ribs meet.

Step 7: Place palm of left hand right above the belly button.

Step 8: Now move the left fingers to the top of the pubic bone.

Step 9: Move the right hand to the base of the tailbone (coccyx).

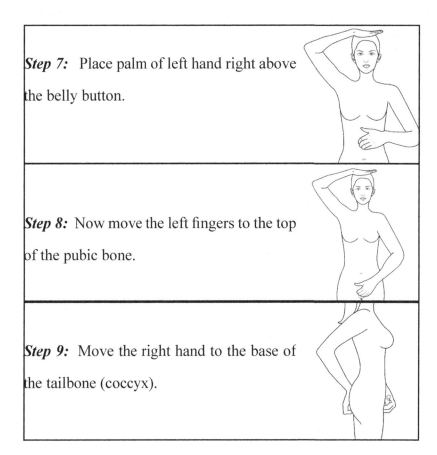

ILLUSTRATION 2
ATTITUDE ADJUSTMENT FLOW

Benefits

- *Aids balancing hormones*

- *Strengthens immune system*

- *Balances emotions*

- *Can help you with insomnia*

	Right	Left
Step 1: Choose a side. Place opposite hand on the chosen side's shoulder so that the palm is resting on top, touching the area between the top tip of shoulder blade and the spine. Then make a ring with the other hand's index fingernail and thumb pad. Have inner knees touching.		
Step 2: Keep the opposite hand on the chosen side's shoulder while making a ring with the other hand's thumb pad and middle fingernail. Inner knees continue touching.		

176

	Right	Left
Step 3: Opposite hand remains on the chosen side's shoulder...but now make a ring with the other hand's thumb pad and ring fingernail. Knees continue touching.		
Step 4: Now make a ring with the thumb pad and the baby fingernail. Note: Inner knees continue touching and opposite hand remains on the shoulder.		

ILLUSTRATION 3
ENERGIZING FLOW

Benefits

- *Fuels you with energy*

- *Focuses your attention*

- *Builds immune system*

- *Helps diminish heavy menstrual cycles*

	Right	*Left*
Step 1: Choose a side. Place same side hand on the inside of the same side foot's arch. The opposite hand goes on the tailbone.		
Step 2: The opposite hand remains on the initial anchoring point on the tailbone, while the same side hand moves up the leg, a hand's-width from the ankle on the inside of the lower leg.		

178

	Right	*Left*
Step 3: Keep anchoring the opposite hand and move the same side hand on the inside just below the knee. (Note: This area is tender for most people unless their diet is really clean.)		
Step 4: The anchor hand on the tail bone remains, and the same side hand moves to the groin area.		
Step 5: The same side hand moves to the opposite side's front ribs while the anchoring hand remains on the tailbone.		

	Right	Left
Step 6: The initial anchor hand moves from the tailbone to the opposite chest point that's just a hand's-width below the collarbone (clavicle).		
Step 7: Now move the initial anchoring hand just below its same side clavicle.		

ILLUSTRATION 4
ANTI-AGING FLOW

Benefits

- *Natural face lift flow*

- *Diminishes mental stress*

- *Helps with digestion (of nutrients/food, life, thoughts, knowledge)*

- *Builds stamina*

- *Helps with a frontal headache*

	Right	*Left*
Step 1: Choose a side. Gently place the opposite hand's fingers on the chosen side's cheek bone in alignment with the edge of its nostril. (This is your anchoring placement for the entire flow.) The same side fingers touch just below the same side clavicle.		
Step2: Now move the same side hand's fingers a hand's-width below the clavicle in alignment with the ears when you are faced straight ahead.		

	Right	*Left*
Step 3: Now move same side fingers to the opposite side's base of the front ribs. Palming this area is recommended.		
Step 4: Place the same side hand to the opposite side's base of the back ribs. Note: It may be easier to use the back of the hand to touch this area.		
Step 5: Place same side hand on the same side base of front ribs.		

	Right	*Left*
Step 6: Place the same side hand on the opposite side of the inner lower thigh (about a hand's-width up from the inner knee).		
Step 7: Place same side hand a hand's-width down from the eye of the opposite knee, just in the hollow space that is on the outside (lateral edge).		
Step 8: Place same side hand on the lateral edge of the opposite calf that is halfway between the knee and the ankle crease.		

	Right	*Left*
Step 9: Sandwich the opposite third toe with the same side fingers.		

ILLUSTRATION 5

DETOXIFYING FLOW

Benefits

- *Helps to detox the body of any toxins, such as alcohol, sugar etc.*

- *Helps diminish back-of-the-head headaches*

- *Great aid for back tension and stress*

- *Can help diminish sciatica (pain shooting down the side of the leg)*

	Right	Left
Step 1: Choose a side. Place opposite hand on the chosen side of the neck. This will be your anchor for the whole flow. Other hand palms the tail bone (coccyx).		
Step2: Now move the hand on the tailbone to its same side sit bone.		

	Right	Left
Step 3: Next move hand from same side sit bone to same side back of the knee.		
Step 4: Place same side hand below and slightly back from its same side lateral (outside) ankle.(in the hollow space there)		
Step 5: Move same side hand from outside ankle to the same side cuboid bone (the lateral edge of the foot just before the toe bones known as metatarsals).		

	Right	Left
Step 6: Now sandwich your same side baby toe with your fingers.		

ABOUT THE AUTHOR, TOMASA MACAPINLAC

With 20 years of experience in Asian Bodywork Therapy blended with her initiation as a Shaman, Tomasa Macapinlac deeply understands why her clients get stuck and teaches them how to create profitable, healthy change so that they look and feel vibrant. Her work brings a unique perspective by blending the physical world with each person's inner guidance.

Tomasa is the creator of several visual and audio guided hands-on healing products, including The Vibrant Energy Flow System, 30 Days to a Vibrant, Healthier, Younger You and her latest – The Basic Cold & Flu Prevention Kit. Her healing work has been enjoyed by people around the world.

In her years before becoming a healer, Tomasa earned a degree in electrical engineering from UC Berkeley. She was an award winning hi-tech salesperson for HP, Motorola, and Windriver (now Intel), drawing upon her people skills while utilizing her electrical engineering knowledge.

Tomasa's infectious laugh and love of hip-hop dance allow her to be fully in her body while leaving an indelible impression on all who meet her. You can find Tomasa and download her free resources at www.selfcarequeendom.com.

Other Resources from Tomasa Macapinlac

THE VIBRANT ENERGY FLOW SYSTEM AUDIO PROGRAM

Audio program (discontinued) that guides you through the five major flows illustrated in this book. Designed to help you overcome exhaustion and have more vitality in your life.

30 DAYS TO A VIBRANT, HEALTHIER, YOUNGER YOU

Video information product that inspired this book and brought in the visual aspect and support around the Vibrant Energy Flow System™. Great for you if you would like to follow along using a video format. Can be purchased at http://www.selfcarequeendom.com/30days.

COLD & FLU PREVENTION KIT

Inspired and designed for clients who find themselves getting a cold or flu more than once per year. Helps to build a healthy immune system and clear out cold or flu bugs quickly. To learn more about this product and to purchase please check out - http://www.selfcarequeendom.com/coldflu.

COMING SOON in 2017!
THE VIBRANT ENERGY FLOW SYSTEM 2.0
HOME STUDY PROGRAM

You can learn about and register for this comprehensive program here -> http://www.selfcarequeendom.com/vefs2-0-offer/.

If you wish to work with Tomasa one-on-one or want her to design a custom program exclusively for you, please send your request with your name, phone number and detailed inquiry in an email to info@selfcarequeendom.com.